Silent Myocardial Ischemia and Infarction

Silent Myocardial Ischemia and Infarction

Second Edition, Revised and Expanded

PETER F. COHN

*Professor of Medicine
and Chief, Cardiology Division
State University of New York
Health Sciences Center at Stony Brook
Stony Brook, New York*

MARCEL DEKKER, INC.   New York and Basel

Library of Congress Cataloging-in-Publication Data

Cohn, Peter F.,
   Silent myocardial ischemia and infarction, 2nd ed. revised and
   expanded
   Includes bibliographies and index.
   1. Silent myocardial ischemia. 2. Heart--Infarction. I. Title. [DNLM:
1. Coronary Disease. 2. Myocardial Infarction. WG 300 C6785s]
RC685.C6C586   1989   616.1'23   88-33532
ISBN 0-8247-8084-1

This book is printed on acid-free paper.

MARCEL DEKKER, INC.
270 Madison Avenue, New York, New York 10016

Current printing (last digit):
10 9 8 7 6 5 4 3

PRINTED IN THE UNITED STATES OF AMERICA

For
my wife, Joan,
and my sons, Alan and Clifford

Preface to the Second Edition

Much has transpired in the field of silent coronary artery disease since the first edition of this book was published in 1986—in fact, enough new data to warrant a second edition. The book is organized as before into six sections, but important new information has been added to all sections, especially in regard to pathophysiology, detection of ischemic episodes with Holter monitoring, results of prognostic studies and last, but certainly not least, additional data on therapeutic interventions for clinicians caring for patients with coronary artery disease. The wealth of new data is attested to by the volume of abstracts presented at the 1986, 1987 and 1988 meetings of the American Heart Association and the American College of Cardiology. It is a matter not only of quantity, but also of quality. *Every* area relating to silent coronary artery disease is now being actively explored by excellent investigators in a multitude of centers. These centers are no longer confined to a few hospitals, as they once were, but are located throughout the United States, Europe and Japan.

Again, I would like to thank the physicians, nurses and medical technicians of the State University of New York Health Sciences Center at Stony Brook for their assistance, with special mention for the superb secretarial work of Mrs. Marlene Landesman.

Peter F. Cohn

Preface to the First Edition

The purpose of this monograph is to discuss what is known—and what is not known—about asymptomatic coronary artery disease and its two major components: silent myocardial ischemia and silent myocardial infarction. These disorders afflict millions of persons, yet little is written about their mechanisms, prognosis, and other characteristics mainly because physicians—and the lay public—traditionally associate myocardial ischemia and infarction with chest pain (or its equivalents). That this is not necessarily so is becoming more and more evident. Symptomatic episodes may represent only the tip of the iceberg of myocardial ischemia.

To evaluate the subject in a systematic way, this book has been organized into five major parts: pathophysiology, prevalence, detection, prognosis, and management of asymptomatic coronary artery disease.

Many of the studies discussed in the following chapters were performed with the assistance of my colleagues at Harvard Medical School and the Brigham and Women's Hospital in Boston, and the State University of

New York Health Sciences Center at Stony Brook. Their contributions are greatly appreciated, as is the expert secretarial assistance of Mrs. Marlene Landesman.

Peter F. Cohn

Contents

Contents

Contents

Silent Myocardial Ischemia and Infarction

Introduction

The realization that not all coronary artery disease must be symptomatic is not a new one, but it has not always received the attention it deserved.

The history of asymptomatic coronary artery disease is basically a history of its two major syndromes—silent myocardial ischemia and silent myocardial infarction. *Silent (painless, asymptomatic) myocardial ischemia* is best defined as objective evidence of transient ischemia (on ECG, radionuclide studies, etc.) in the absence of angina or its usual equivalents. *Silent (unrecognized) myocardial infarction* is essentially an ECG diagnosis. Autopsy reports of extensive coronary disease in persons apparently free of symptoms were the first important clues to the existence of this syndrome [1]. The next important—although indirect—milestones were studies of unexpected sudden death in which large numbers of previously asymptomatic persons were involved. But it was not until patients with coronary artery disease were actually observed to be free of pain during episodes of transient myocardial ischemia on exercise tests [2,3] and during ambulatory electrocardiographic monitoring [4] that interest in this subject increased [5].

1

My own interest in asymptomatic coronary artery disease began in the early 1970s and initially involved ECG responses during exercise testing. Our first study was reported at the American Heart Association meetings in 1975 [6] and was followed by a review in 1977 [7] which described the unexpectedly vast scope of the disorder. Introduction of the concept of a "defective anginal warning system" soon followed with speculation as to its causes and effect on prognosis [8]. It became apparent to me that if this subject were to be investigated fully, a classification system for asymptomatic coronary artery disease was necessary. Accordingly, in 1981 [9], we proposed that silent myocardial ischemia be thought of as occurring in three types of patients with coronary artery disease (Table 1). The first group consisted of persons who were totally asymptomatic and the second group of persons who were asymptomatic after an infarction. In addition, silent myocardial ischemia can be seen in patients with angina who also have asymptomatic episodes. The key to this classification is in documentation of active ischemia; persons who have asymptomatic coronary artery disease but are not experiencing active ischemia are purposely not involved in this classification. Thus, someone with an infarction, a totally occluded vessel and no ongoing ischemia by objective criteria would be excluded.

The five major questions that were posed in the 1981 review [9] are still pertinent today and form the basis for this monograph, slightly modified. They are

1. What is the pathophysiologic basis of silent myocardial ischemia and silent myocardial infarction?
2. What is the prevalence of the different types of silent myocardial ischemia, and of silent myocardial infarction?
3. What are the most reliable noninvasive methods of detecting the syndrome of silent myocardial ischemia, and what are the indications for cardiac catheterization in asymptomatic persons?
4. What is the prognosis of patients with silent myocardial ischemia and/or silent myocardial infarction?

Table 1   Types of Cases in Which Silent Myocardial Ischemia May Be Found

I. In persons who are totally asymptomatic
II. In persons who are asymptomatic following a myocardial infarction, but still demonstrate active ischemia
III. In persons with angina who are asymptomatic with some episodes of myocardial ischemia, but not others

5. How should silent myocardial ischemia be treated if at all? Others have also posed similar questions [10].

The first attempt of answering these questions in a systematic way was in a seminar that appeared in 1983 in the Journal of the American College of Cardiology [11]. This was followed by the first international symposium on Silent Myocardial Ischemia held in Geneva, Switzerland, in 1984 under the auspices of the European Society of Cardiology [12]. Numerous other national and international symposia have been held since then. In 1986 the first edition of this monograph was published [13] and was soon joined by several other important state-of-the-art publications [14-16]. In addition to these publications, there have been three other articles that should have special interest for readers of this book. These are the reports of the combined American College of Cardiology/American Heart Association Task Force on Assessment of Diagnostic and Therapeutic Cardiovascular Procedures on exercise testing [17], coronary angioplasty [18], and Holter monitoring [19]. Each report contains a section on the indications for these procedures in (1) asymptomatic patients at high risk for latent coronary artery disease, and/or (2) those patients with symptoms but in whom silent ischemia is suspected or has been demonstrated.

REFERENCES

1. M. D. Roseman. Painless myocardial infarction: A review of the literature and analysis of 220 cases. *Ann. Intern. Med., 41*:1 (1954).

2. A. M. Master and A. M. Geller. The extent of completely asymptomatic coronary artery disease. *Am. J. Cardiol., 23*:173 (1969).

3. V. F. Froelicher, F. G. Yanowitz, and A. J. Thompson. The correlation of coronary angiography and the electrocardiographic response to maximal treadmill testing in 76 asymptomatic men. *Circulation, 48*:597 (1973).

4. S. Stern and D. Tzivoni. Early detection of silent ischaemic heart disease by 24-hour electrocardiographic monitoring of active subjects. *Br. Heart J., 35*: 481 (1974).

5. L. S. Gettes. Painless myocardial ischemia. *Chest, 66*:612 (1974).

6. H. E. Lindsey and P. F. Cohn. "Silent" ischemia during and after exercise testing in patients with coronary artery disease (abstr). *Circulation, 52*(Suppl 11):46 (1975).

7. P. F. Cohn. Severe asymptomatic coronary artery disease: A diagnostic, prognostic and therapeutic puzzle. *Am. J. Med., 62*:565 (1977).

8. P. F. Cohn. Silent myocardial ischemia in patients with a defective anginal warning system. *Am. J. Cardiol., 45*:697 (1980).

9. P. F. Cohn. Asymptomatic coronary artery disease: Pathophysiology, diagnosis, management. *Mod. Concepts Cardiovasc. Dis., 50*:55 (1981).

10. A. S. Iskandrian, B. L. Segal, and G. S. Anderson. Asymptomatic myocardial ischemia. *Arch. Intern. Med., 141*:95 (1981).

11. P. F. Cohn. Introduction to Seminar on Asymptomatic Coronary Artery Disease. *J. Am. Coll. Cardiol., 3*:922 (1983).

12. W. Rutishauser and H. Roskamm, eds. *Silent Myocardial Ischemia.* Springer-Verlag, Berlin, 1984.

13. P. F. Cohn. *Silent Myocardial Ischemia and Infarction.* Marcel Dekker, New York, 1986.

14. C. J. Pepine, ed. *Cardiology Clinics: Silent Myocardial Ischemia.* W. B. Saunders, Philadelphia, 1986.

15. P. F. Cohn and W. Kannel, eds. Recognition, pathogenesis and management options in silent coronary artery disease. *Circulation, 75*(Suppl II):1-54 (1987).

16. T. von Arnim and A. Maseri, eds. *Silent Ischemia: Current Concepts and Management.* Steinkopff, Darmstadt (1987).

17. R. C. Schlant, C. G. Blomqvist, R. O. Brandenburg, et al. A report of the American College of Cardiology/American Heart Association Task Force on Assessment of Diagnostic and Therapeutic Cardiovascular Procedures: Guidelines on Exercise Testing. *J. Am. Coll. Cardiol., 8*:725 (1986).

18. T. J. Ryan, D. P. Faxon, R. M. Gunnar, et al. A Report of the American College of Cardiology/American Heart Association Task Force on Assessment of Diagnostic and Therapeutic Cardiovascular Procedures: Guidelines on Percutaneous Transluminal Coronary Angioplasty. *J. Am. Coll. Cardiol., 12*:529 (1988).

19. S. B. Knoebel, M. H. Crawford, M. I. Dunn, et al. A Report of the American College of Cardiology/American Heart Association Task Force on Assessment of Diagnostic and Therapeutic Cardiovascular Procedures: Guidelines for Clinical Use of Ambulatory Electrocardiography. *J. Am. Coll. Cardiol. 13*:249 (1989).

I
PATHOPHYSIOLOGY OF SILENT MYOCARDIAL ISCHEMIA

1

Cardiac Pain Mechanisms

Because pain is subjective, it cannot be easily investigated with the kinds of experimental models that are usually employed in laboratory settings. In those experimental pain studies that can be performed, some pain modalities are easier to assess than others. Somatic pain is one of the "easier" types, whereas visceral pain is harder to categorize experimentally. Therefore, cardiac pain, being visceral in nature, does not lend itself easily to reproducible studies in the animal laboratory.

I. NEUROANATOMY OF CARDIAC PAIN PATHWAYS

What has been established in the animal laboratory is the gross anatomy of the apparent cardiac nociceptive pathways. The afferent fibers that run in the cardiac sympathetic nerves are usually thought of as the essential pathway for the transmission of cardiac pain. The atria and ventricles are abundantly supplied with sympathetic sensory innervation; from the heart the sensory nerve endings connect to afferent fibers in cardiac nerve bundles which in turn connect to the upper five thoracic sympathetic ganglia and the upper five thoracic dorsal roots of the spinal cord (Figure 1). Recent reexamination of the extrinsic cardiac veins and ganglia by Janes and colleagues [1] suggests that the anatomic pattern of the innervation of the human heart is not as unique as traditionally defined (i.e., consisting of three major sympathetic cardiac nerves and ganglia). Instead, Janes and colleagues found the pattern to be very similar to that in other animals, especially the baboon. Within the spinal cord itself, impulses mediated by this sympathetic afferent route probably converge with impulses from somatic thoracic structures onto the same ascending spinal neurons. The contribution of cells of the spirothalamic tract have been studied extensively by Foreman and colleagues [2,3]. This would be the basis for cardiac referred pain, i.e., pain referred to the chest, wall, arm, back, etc. In addition to this "convergence-projection theory" (first proposed by Ruch [4] over 30 years ago and more recently supported by Foreman's studies), the contribution of vagal afferent fibers must be acknowledged or else we have no explanation for cardiac pain referred to the jaw and neck. How these vagal fibers are activated remains unclear.

II. THEORIES OF CARDIAC PAIN

The links between disease of the coronary arteries and cardiac pain go back to the time of Heberden's original descriptions of the clinical picture of angina pectoris. Early writers believed that coronary spasm was common and that interruption in blood supply could produce pain. Lewis [5] has noted that Potain was the first to draw the analogy between pain arising from ischemic myocardium and an ischemic limb. But what was the actual "trigger" that stimulated the sensory nerve endings? Lewis proposed that a chemical pain stimulus was involved, the so-called "factor P" produced by exercise-induced ischemia. Others proposed that anoxia itself was the cause of the pain. The "trigger" is still unclear. In the last several years, there has been increasing attention to the role of peptides

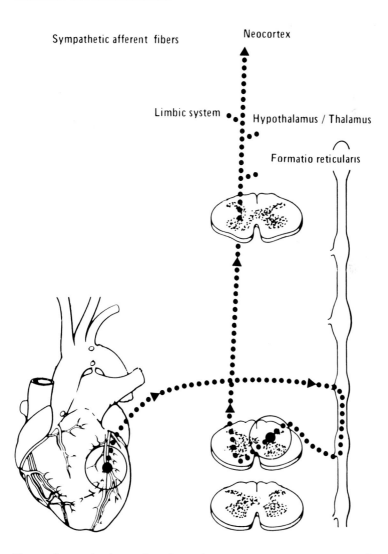

Figure 1 Mechanisms of cardiac pain. (From C. Droste and H. Roskamm, in *Silent Myocardial Ischemia* [W. Rutishauser and H. Roskamm, eds.], Springer-Verlag, Berlin, 1984.)

in cardiac innervation [6]. Distributed throughout cardiac and extra cardiac nerves, they may be acting alone or in combination with classical adrenergic and cholinergic transmitters. At one time, a mechanical stimulus (stretching of the coronary arteries) was also proposed as the cause of the pain even when ischemia itself was not induced. This was suggested after watching the behavior of laboratory animals whose coronary arteries were stretched.

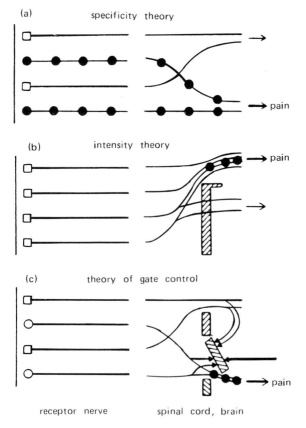

Figure 2 Theories of neural encoding of peripheral painful stimuli. (From C. Droste, H. Roskamm. In *Silent Ischemia: Current Concepts and Management.* [T. von Arnim, A. Maseri, eds.]. Steinkopff, Darmstadt, 1987, p. 27.)

Recently, the nociceptive (pain-bearing) function of the cardiac sympathetic fibers has itself been challenged, especially by Malliani [7-9]. Malliani notes that the two main hypotheses for the peripheral (somatic) manifestation of pain are the "intensity" and "specificity" hypotheses (Figure 2). The "intensity" hypothesis assumes that pain results from an excessive stimulation of receptive structures. The "specificity" hypothesis postulates that pain is conceived as a specific sensation by excitation of a well-defined nociceptive system that responds to noxious stimuli. Malliani poses the question: Do specific cardiac nociceptors exist? Are there really hundreds of cardiac nerve fibers exclusively designed for signaling higher centers about certain kinds of coronary emergencies? Another theory, of neuronal encoding of peripheral painful stimuli states that pain is felt as a result of an imbalance between different diameter fibers and central impulses. An element of inhibition is present in this schema (the "gate control" theory), most likely within the posterior horn of the spinal cord (Figure 3) [10].

III. EXPERIMENTAL STUDIES

Electrophysiologic studies of the afferent fibers that are most likely to convey cardiac nociception (the ventricular fibers) evaluated these fibers

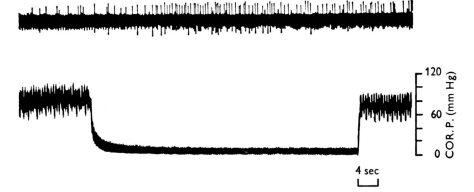

Figure 3 Effect of myocardial ischemia on an afferent unit in the inferior cardiac nerve. The sudden fall in coronary pressure (Cor. P. in mmHg) occurred when the inflow was stopped. There was some background activity which showed a marked increase during ischemia. (From A.M. Brown and A. Malliani, *J. Physiol.,* *212*:685, 1971.)

for absence of spontaneous impulse activity, unresponsiveness to normal physiologic hemodynamic stimuli, and the ability to respond to stimuli of pathophysiologic significance. In Malliani's experiments, multifiber recordings were obtained from afferent sympathetic fibers. As indicated in Figure 3, excitation could be demonstrated during interruption of coronary blood flow. In the early experiments, recruitment of a few silent units, i.e., with obvious background discharge, could be demonstrated by computer assisted techniques. This recruitment suggested to Malliani

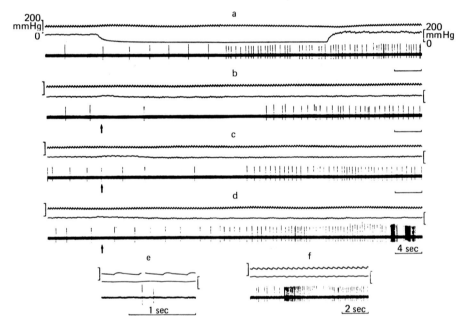

Figure 4   Activity of an afferent sympathetic unmyelinated nerve fiber with a left ventricular ending. Tracings represent from top to bottom: systemic arterial pressure, coronary perfusion pressure, nerve impulse activity (cathode-ray oscilloscope recordings). (a) Interruption of the left main coronary artery perfusion; (b) intracoronary administration, beginning at the arrow, of bradykinin 5 ng/kg; (c) intracoronary administration of bradykinin 10 ng/kg; (d) intracoronary administration of bradykinin 30 ng/kg; (e) electrical stimulation of the left inferior cardiac nerve activating the affering fiber to calculate the conduction velocity; (f) mechanical probing, marked by a bar, of an area of the external surface of the left ventricle. (From F. Lombardi, P. Della Bella, R. Casati, and A. Malliani. *Circ. Res.*, *48*:69, 1981. Reproduced with the permission of the American Heart Association.)

and co-workers that specific cardiac nociceptors were present. Reexamination of the data in later experiments [8] cast doubts about this interpretation in light of the animal preparation used. In the preparation, the spinal cord was transsected and the baseline arterial pressure was low enough to "artificially" reduce the normal background discharge of the fibers. In other experiments [11] using coronary occlusion or the intracoronary administration of bradykinin—a naturally occurring substance that is believed to play a role in the genesis of cardiac pain—no recruitment of silent afferent units could be demonstrated (Figure 4). Thus, whether myelinated or not, the ventricular afferent fibers always possessed some degree of spontaneous impulse activity and a responsiveness to normal hemodynamic stimuli. Malliani concluded that the sensitivity to both mechani-

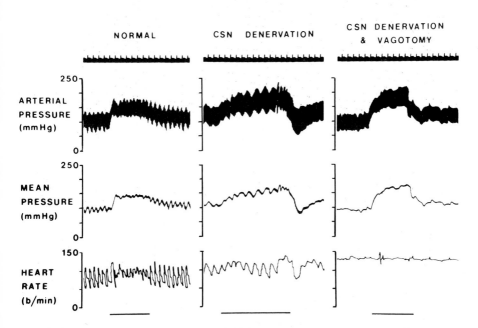

Figure 5   Reflex effects of aortic distension (indicated by the bottom bars) on systemic arterial pressure and heart rate in a conscious dog. The left panel depicts the control response, the middle panel the response after carotid sinoaortic denervation and the right panel the response after further sectioning of both vagi. Note the progressive increase of the pressor response that follows the denervation procedures. "Pain" (i.e., agitation, etc.) was not observed in any of these experiments. (From M. Pagani, P. Pizzinelli, M. Bergamaschi, and A. Malliani. *Circ. Res., 50*:125, 1982.)

cal and chemical stimuli, such as bradykinin, was not unique, as others [12] claimed.

Malliani has also commented on behavior of conscious animals exposed to intense excitation of cardiovascular sympathetic fibers. In one of his experiments, the thoracic aorta was stretched via an implanted and inflatable rubber cylinder [13]. A mechanical stimulus elicited a pressor reflex without any pain. In the other experiment, bradykinin was injected directly into a branch of the left coronary artery that had previously been cannulated. Despite pressor responses, there was no pain (Figure 5). However, when the same experiment was performed 3 days after surgery, the animal was obviously in pain; the surgery had "facilitated" the cardiac pain. Under chronic conditions with an implanted occluder, Theroux et al. [14] reported pain responses are variable. Thus, as noted earlier, Malliani has concluded that no specific cardiac nociceptive apparatus could be confirmed. Rather, the "intensity" hypothesis appears a more valid explanation, especially a modified version that is based on a unique spatiotemporal pattern of afferent discharges with central inhibitory modulation [15].

IV. RELATION OF EXPERIMENTAL STUDIES TO THE CLINICAL SETTING

How does the "intensity" pain mechanism relate to the clinical setting and particularly to the occurrence of silent myocardial ischemia? Sufficient levels of afferent impulses must be reached and an appropriate activation of the central ascending pathway must be established before a breakthrough can occur and there is a conscious perception of pain. The level of impulses may be influenced by hypertension and tachycardia preceding the ischemia episodes—the more general the cardiac sympathetic afferent discharge, the more likely the intensity of discharges will reach the critical threshold necessary to convert a receptive process (nociception) into a conscious experience (angina pectoris). By not reaching this critical threshold, ischemia remains "silent." This is not the only mechanism possible. For example, after a transmural myocardial infarction, Barber et al. [16] showed areas of both sympathetic and vagal afferent "autodenervation" produced apical to the infarcted region. Ischemia can have the same effect [17].

V. CONCLUSIONS

The neurophysiology of the cardiac pain pathway continues to be an enigma and the link between pain and cardiac tissue damage remains elusive.

REFERENCES

1. R. D. Janes, J. C. Brandys, D. A. Hopkins, D. E. Johnstone, D. A. Murphy, and J. A. Armour. Anatomy of human extrinsic cardiac nerves and ganglia. *Am. J. Cardiol., 57*:299 (1986).

2. R. D. Foreman, C. A. Ohata, and K. D. Gerhard. Neural mechanisms underlying cardiac pain. In *Neural Mechanisms in Cardiac Arrhythmias* (P. J. Schwartz, A. M. Brown, A. Malliani, and A. Zanchetti, eds.), Raven Press, New York, 1978, p. 191.

3. R. D. Foreman. Spinal substrates of visceral pain. In *Spinal Afferent Processing* (T. L. Yaksh, ed.). Plenum Press, New York, 1986, p. 217.

4. T. C. Ruch. Pathophysiology of pain. In *A Textbook of Physiology* (J. F. Fulton, ed.), W.B. Saunders Co., Philadelphia, 1955, p. 358.

5. T. Lewis. Pain in muscular ischemia: Its relation to anginal pain. *Arch. Intern. Med., 49*:713 (1932).

6. E. Weihe. Peripheral innervation of the heart. In *Silent Ischemia: Current Concepts and Management* (T. von Arnim, A. Maseri, eds.). Steinkopff, Darmstadt, 1987, p. 9.

7. A. Malliani and F. Lombardi. Consideration of the fundamental mechanisms eliciting cardiac pain. *Am. Heart J., 103*:575 (1982).

8. A. Malliani. Cardiovascular sympathetic afferent fibers. *Rev. Physiol. Biochem. Pharmacol., 94*:11 (1982).

9. A. Malliani. The elusive link between transient myocardial ischemia and pain. *Circulation, 73*:201 (1986).

10. C. Droste and H. Roskamm. Experimental approach to painful and painless ischemia. In *Silent Ischemia: Current Concepts and Management.* (T. von Arnim, A. Maseri, eds.). Steinkopff, Darmstadt, 1987, p. 27.

11. F. Lombardi, P. Dell Bella, R. Casati, and A. Malliani. Effects of intracoronary administration of bradykinin on the impulse activity of afferent sympathetic unmyelinated fibers with left ventreicular endings in the cat. *Circ. Res., 48*:69 (1981).

12. D. G. Baker, H. M. Coleridge, J. C. G. Coleridge, and T. Terndrum. Search for a cardiac nociceptor: Stimulation by bradykinin of sympathetic afferent nerve endings in the heart of the cat. *J. Physiol., 306*:519 (1980).

13. M. Pagani, P. Pizzinelli, M. Bergamaschi, and A. Malliani. A positive feedback sympathetic pressor reflex during stretch of the thoracic aorta in conscious dogs. *Circ. Res., 50*:125 (1982).

14. P. Theroux, J. Ross, D. Franklin, W. S. Kemper, and S. Sassayama. Regional myocardial function in the conscious dog during acute coronary occlusion and responses to morphine, propranolol, nitroglycerin, and lidocaine. *Circulation, 53*:302 (1976).

15. A. Malliani. Pathophysiology of ischemic cardiac pain. In *Silent Ischemia: Current Concepts and Management.* (T. von Arnim, A. Maseri, eds.). Seinkopff, Darmstadt, 1987, p. 21.

16. M. J. Barber, T. M. Mueller, B. G. Davies, R. M. Gill, and D. P. Zipes. Interruption of sympathetic and vagal-mediated afferent responses by transmural myocardial infarction. *Circulation, 72*:623 (1985).

17. H. Inoue, B. T. Skale and D. P. Zipes. Effects of ischemia on cardiac afferent sympathetic and vagal reflexes in dogs. *Am. J. Physiol., 255 (Heart Circ. Physiol., 24)*:H26 (1988).

2

Alterations in Sensitivity to Pain in Patients with Silent Myocardial Ischemia

Why pain is not present during episodes of silent myocardial ischemia is unclear; one possible mechanism is an alteration in the patient's sensibility to pain, either centrally or peripherally.

I. STUDIES OF PAIN THRESHOLD AND PAIN PERCEPTION

The most thorough series of investigations of this subject to date has been that of Droste and Roskamm. In their first study [1], these investigators reported results in 42 men (mean age 51 years). All patients had angiographically confirmed coronary artery disease, i.e., $\geq 75\%$ stenosis in at least one major coronary artery. In addition, they all had >1.0 mm ST segment depression on multiple exercise studies. Patients were divided into two groups depending on the occurrence of angina pectoris during the exercise tests. Factors such as digitalis medication, hypokalemia, valvular heart disease, etc., that could have been responsible for specious ST segment depression were excluded. All patients had normal neurologic examinations. There were 20 patients in the asymptomatic group; 16 had ECG evidence of prior infarction, but only six had pain with the infarction. Furthermore, 16 of the patients had no angina during everyday activity; the other five had complained of pain in the past. By contrast, in

Table 1   Comparison of Selected Medical Variables Measured in Patients with Symptomatic and Asymptomatic Myocardial Ischemia

	Myocardial ischemia			
	Symptomatic (n = 22)		Asymptomatic (n = 20)	
1-vessel disease	9		3	
2-vessel disease	3	2.1 ± 0.9	3	2.5 ± 0.8
3-vessel disease	10		14	
Friesinger score	8.6 ± 3.1		10.4 ± 2.6	
Ejection fraction (%)	60 ± 16		58 ± 12	
Heart volume (ml)	816 ± 142		856 ± 220	
Heart volume related to body weight (ml/kg)	10.9 ± 1.2		11.1 ± 2.5	
Previous myocardial infarction (no. of patients)	17		16	
Risk factors				
Age (yr)	51 ± 5.8		52 ± 9.6	
Smoking	17		10	
Hypertension ($>140 > 95$ mmHg)	8		8	
Diabetes	1		2	
Cholesterol (mg/dl)	240 ± 40		237 ± 65	
Triglycerides (mg/dl)	195 ± 83		174 ± 79	

All data are = standard deviation values.
Differences between the symptomatic and asymptomatic groups for each variable were not significant.
Source: C. Droste and H. Roskamm. Experimental pain measurement in patients with asymptomatic myocardial ischemia. *J. Am. Coll. Cardiol.*, 1:940, 1983.

the symptomatic group (22 patients), only 2 of 17 patients who had prior infarctions had no pain with the infarctions. Distribution of coronary risk factors was similar in both groups, as were angiographic features (Table 1).

Droste and Roskamm studied three different modalities of pain perception. The first was an electrical pain threshold test in which the magnitude of pain current applied to the thigh was evaluated. The value of threshold was reported according to the degree of electrical current used (in mA). The second test was a standard cold pressor test in which patient's left arm was submerged in water cooled to 4 °C. The third test was a modified form of the submaximal effort tourniquet technique in which the working muscle of the left arm is stressed. The end point in the first test was the actual amount of electrical current needed to produce pain. In the other two tests, the time that elapsed before the patient perceived pain,

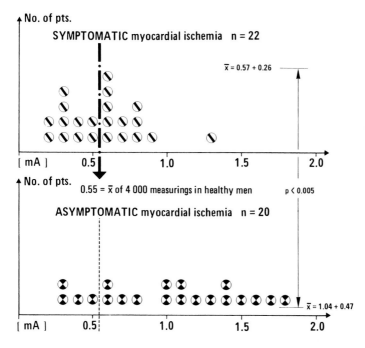

Figure 1 Electrical pain threshold in symptomatic and asymptomatic patients. (From C. Drose and H. Roskamm. *J. Am. Coll. Cardiol.*, *1*:940, 1983.)

or was no longer able to tolerate pain, was measured. The results of these studies showed striking differences when the two groups were compared. For example, when pain threshold was determined, symptomatic patients demonstrated a mean electrical pain threshold of 0.57 mA (Figure 1, top). This finding is in agreement with other studies performed in healthy men in which 0.55 mA was the average value. Asymptomatic patients had a much wider range of values with a mean value of 1.04 mA (Figure 1, bottom). During the cold pressor tests, asymptomatic patients showed much greater values for pain tolerance than did symptomatic patients (Figure 2,

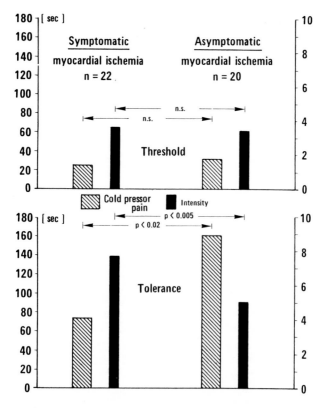

Figure 2 Cold pressor test: group differences for threshold and tolerance levels. (Hatched columns = stimulus intensity; solid columns = subjective experience of pain). (From C. Droste and H. Roskamm. *J. Am. Coll. Cardiol., 1*:940, 1983.)

bottom). Pain thresholds showed a similar trend, but the differences were not statistically significant. During the arm muscle ischemic pain rest, asymptomatic patients had a higher pain threshold and pain tolerance than symptomatic patients, though only the latter difference achieved statistical significance. In addition, asymptomatic patients rated a strong stimulus as actually being less intense than did the symptomatic patients. (This was also true in the cold pressor test.) In later studies, measurements of transcutaneous partial oxygen tension in the occluded forearm were added [2]. This allowed information about oxygen supply and demand in the resting and working muscle to be obtained and the development of ischemia and anoxia quantitatively assessed. This is depicted in Figure 3, in which asymptomatic patients exhibited lower oxygen tensions at threshold

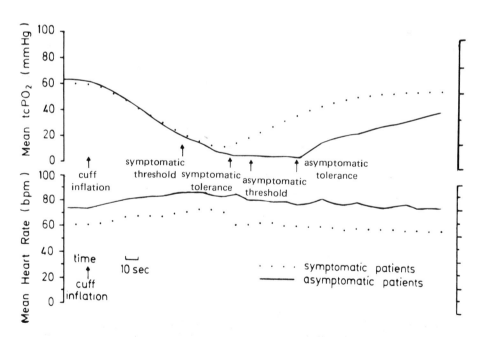

Figure 3 Time course of mean values of transcutaneous partial oxygen tension (tcpO₂) (upper traces) and heart rate (lower traces) for symptomatic (dashed lines; n = 6) and asymptomatic (solid lines; n = 6) patients. Time of cuff inflation denoted by arrows. Threshold and tolerance levels are depicted separately (arrows) for symptomatic and asymptomatic groups. (From C. Droste, M. W. Greenlee, and H. Roskamm. *Pain, 26*:199, 1986.)

(a) Threshold values

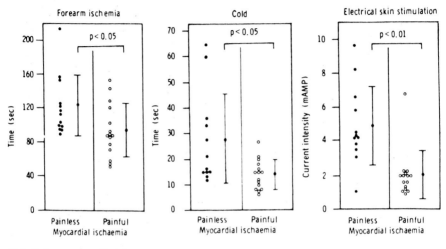

(b) Tolerance values

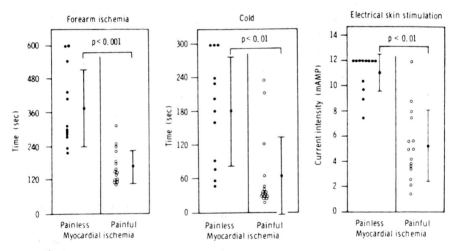

Figure 4   Threshold (a) and tolerance (b) values for a variety of painful stimuli in the 2 study patient groups. Although both threshold and tolerance values were, on average, greater in the patients with painless ischemia, overlap between the 2 groups was considerable. (From J. J. Glazier, S. Chierchia, M. J. Brown, and A. Maseri. *Am. J. Cardiol., 58*:667, 1986.)

and tolerance that symptomatic patients and needed more time to reach these levels.

The pain threshold studies of Droste and Roskamm were subsequently confirmed by Glazier et al. [3]. They studied 27 patients, 12 with predominantly painless ischemia and 15 with predominantly painful ischemia. Threshold and tolerance value were greater in the painless group, but overlap was considerable (Figure 4). Using a different pain test, electrical dental pulp stimulation, Falcone et al. were able to show a significant difference in pain threshold between patients with and without painless ischemia [4].

II. CLINICAL FEATURES THAT MAY EXPLAIN ABSENCE OF PAIN

Droste and Roskamm evaluated three arguments put forth as possible explanations for the lack of pain. The first has to do with destruction of nociceptive pathways by infarction, diffuse ischemia or some type of neuropathy. In these patients, however, the frequency of myocardial infarctions, extensive multivessel disease, diabetes or alcoholism was similar in both the symptomatic and asymptomatic subgroups. The authors maintained that only radical surgical procedures—transplantation, autotransplantation, plexectomy—could sufficiently denervate a heart so that angina became absent. The authors also felt that their study amply demonstrated that the intensity of ischemia is not necessarily reduced in asymptomatic patients. They based this on the finding that the degree of ischemia—as determined by ST depression—was comparable in both groups. (We comment further on this factor—the amount of myocardium at jeopardy—in Chapter 4.) Thus, they concluded that the hyposensibility to pain in general that they reported best differentiated the asymptomatic from the symptomatic patients. This supported earlier, less quantitative data from studies of patients with silent myocardial infarction [5].*

The authors then posed the question as to which mechanisms were involved in the decreased sensibility to pain: pain-discriminating ability versus individual response tendencies that categorize a stimulus as pain. The authors felt that some of their data, especially that dealing with the differences in electrically determined pain thresholds and thresholds for ischemic pain, supported the former mechanism. But the tendency for

---

*Pain mechanisms in silent myocardial infarctions are discussed further in Chapter 7.

asymptomatic patients to rate painful stimuli as less intense—and thus tolerate the stimulus much longer—argues also for a difference in response tendencies. The two factors are not necessarily independ;ent of each other.

III. POSSIBLE ROLE OF ENDORPHINS

Could endorphic mechanisms influence the difference in pain responses? Normally, varying concentrations of these opioidlike substances exist in plasma and cerebrospinal fluid and may be important in mediating pain sensitivity [6]. VanRijn and Rabkin [7] reported that injection of the opioid-antagonist naloxone precipiated angina earlier during exercise-induced ischemia than a placebo. However, they only tested five patients. We were unable to reproduce these results in eight symptomatic patients, nor were we able to use this agent to precipitate angina during treadmill exercise tests in nine patients with documented silent myocardial ischemia [8]. In a similar study, Ellestad and Kuan [9] reported on their findings in 10 men with asymptomatic but positive stress tests. These men were given naloxone, 2 mg intravenously, and the tests repeated. No chest pain was reported by any patient and naloxone did not significantly alter exercise duration, heart rate, blood pressure, or ST segment changes compared to the control test.

Droste and Roskamm have reported results different from those cited above. They studied 60 patients [10] in a manner similar to their earlier studies in 42 patients [1]. The 60 patients were evenly divided between those with and those without asymptomatic ischemia. The asymptomatic patients had reproducible symptomatic manifestations of myocardial ischemia in several exercise tests. Mean ST depression was 3.8 mm (0.38 mV). Factors that could have indicated false-positive ST segment depression (such as other forms of heart disease or cardiac medications) were excluded. Most of these patients did not have angina during everyday activities and many had had prior myocardial infarctions. All patients had angiographically proven coronary artery disease. A control group of 30 patients with symptomatic coronary artery disease had less ST segment depression during exercise testing (mean 2.2 mm), but other selected mechanical variables showed no difference between the two groups. These variables included age, smoking history and other clinical features, as well as angiographic measurements such as number of vessels diseased, ejection fraction, etc. The three different pain-receptive modalities employed in their previous studies were repeated in this study with similar results. In 10 asymptomatic patients, the tests were repeated following intravenous injection of 2 mg of naloxone and again after a placebo injection. There were no differences in parameters of exercise testing (maximum effort, heart rate, blood pressure, or ST segment depression) between the placebo tests and those employing naloxone. Two of the ten patients developed angina during the naloxone test, though one required 4 mg of the drug before this response was elicited. The most striking finding occurred during the ischemic pain test in which arm ischemia is produced by a tourniquet. Both the threshold to pain and tolerance to it were significantly altered after naloxone administration (Figure 4). The investigators concluded that the results lent support to their previous work showing a differential sensitivity to pain and suggested a possible role for endorphic mechanisms

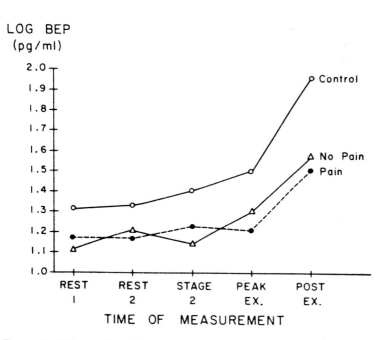

Figure 5 Effects of exercise on plasma beta-endorphin levels in control subjects and patients with silent myocardial ischemia (no pain) or symptomatic ischemia (pain). Beta-endorphin levels are the logarithmic transformation of the original data. Values are group means. Stage 2 = approximately 6 min of exercise; Peak Ex = peak exercise; Post Ex = 10 min after exercise. (From G. V. Heller, C. W. Garber, M. J. Connolly, C. F. Allen-Rowlands, S. F. Siconolfi, D. S. Gann, and R. A. Carleton. *Am. J. Cardiol., 59*:735, 1987.)

Table 2 Postexercise Endorphin Levels Versus Anginal Status

Age (yr) and sex	Cath CAD	History of MI	Time to angina (sec)	Pos RNV	Rest EF (%)	Exercise-induced ST↓	Angina	Post-exercise endorphin level
73M	0	+	140	+	72	+	+	8.3
64M	+	+	255	+	47	+	+	3.7
68M	+	+	...	+	58	+	0	19.5
56M	+	+	230	0	24	0	0	3.2
55M	0	0	...	+	75	+	+	7.3
63M	0	+	...	0	56	0	0	4.5
53F	+	0	375	0	56	+	+	3.5
43M	0	+	...	0	62	+	0	7.0
61M	0	+	270	+	62	+	+	5.9
36M	0	0	...	0	59	+	0	4.5
61M	+	+	192	+	51	+	+	13.0
64M	+	+	...	0	51	+	0	5.0
56F	0	0	200	0	61	+	+	7.1
58F	0	0	...	+	71	0	0	11.8
58M	0	0	267	+	49	0	+	3.2
67M	+	+	200	+	41	+	+	1.5
40F	+	+	180	+	62	+	+	11.5
64F	+	+	80	+	40	0	+	1.3
75F	0	0	...	+	72	+	0	8.5
67M	0	+	...	+	56	+	0	12.5
73M	+	0	130	0	59	+	+	0.0
60M	+	+	...	+	59	+	0	5.8
57M	0	0	585	0	57	+	+	2.6
61M	+	+	625	0	48	0	+	11.9
66F	+	+	120	+	47	+	+	2.6

CAD = coronary artery disease; Cath = catheterized; EF = ejection fraction; MI = myocardial infarction; RNV = radionuclide ventriculogram; ST↓ = ST-segment depression; + = present; 0 = absent.
Source: D. S. Sheps, K. F. Adams, A. Hinderliter, C. Price, J. Bissette, G. Orlando, B. Bargolis, and G. Koch. *Am. J. Cardiol., 59*:523, 1987.

in silent myocardial ischemia. Several papers from different laboratories have dealt directly with this issue, i.e., via measurements of plasma endorphin levels. The study of Glazier et al. cited earlier found similar levels in symptomatic and asymptomatic ischemia. This was confirmed by two other studies (Figure 5) [11,12]. The study of Sheps et al. [13], however, does suggest a causative role for endorphins but even in this study, there was considerable overlap (Table 2). Higher levels were also reported by

Falcone et al. [14] in patients with silent infarction, as well as those with silent ischemia.

In summary, the evidence linking endorphins to silent myocardial ischemia is at best inconclusive.

IV. CONCLUSIONS

There is evidence to suggest that some patients with silent myocardial ischemia have an altered sensibility to certain types of pain. It is not clear whether endorphins influence this hyposensibility.

REFERENCES

1. C. Droste and H. Roskamm. Experimental pain measurement in patients with asymptomatic myocardial ischemia. *J. Am. Coll. Cardiol., 1*:940 (1983).

2. C. Droste, M. W. Greenlee, and H. Roskamm. A defective angina pectoris warning system: Experimental findings of ischemic and electrical pain test. *Pain, 26*:199 (1986).

3. J. J. Glazier, S. Chierchia, M. J. Brown, and A. Maseri. Importance of generalized defective perception of painful stimuli as a cause of silent myocardial ischemia in chronic stable angina pectoris. *Am. J. Cardiol., 58*:667 (1986).

4. C. Falcone, R. Sconocchia, L. Guasti, S. Codega, C. Montemartini, and G. Specchia. Dental pain threshold and angina pectoris in patients with coronary artery disease. *J. Am. Coll. Cardiol., 12*:348 (1988).

5. P. Procacei, M. Zoppi, L. Padeletii, and M. Maresca. Myocardial infarction without pain. A study of the sensory function of the upper limbs. *Pain, 2*:309 (1976).

6. M. S. Buchsbaum, G. C. Davies, R. Coppola, and D. Naber. Opiate pharmacology and individual differences. I. Phychophysical pain measurements. *Pain, 10*:367 (1981).

7. T. VanRijn and S. W. Rabkin. Effect of naloxone, a specific opioid antagonist, on exercise induced angina pectoris (Abstr). *Circulation, 65*(Suppl 4):149 (1981).

8. P. F. Cohn, R. Patcha, S. Singh, S. C. Vlay, G. Mallis, and W. Lawson. Effect of naloxone on exercise tests in patients with symptomatic and silent myocardial ischemia (abstr). *Clin. Res., 33*:177A (1985).

9. M. H. Ellestad and P. Kuan. Naloxone and asymptomatic ischemia. Failure to induce angina during exercise testing. *Am. J. Cardiol., 54*:928 (1984).

10. C. Droste and H. Roskamm. Pain measurement and pain modification by naloxone in patients with asymptomatic myocardial ischemia. In *Silent Myo-*

cardial Ischemia (W. Rutischauser and H. Roskamm, eds.), Springer-Verlag, Berlin, 1984, pp. 14-23.

11. F. Weidinger, A. Hammerle, H. Sochor, R. Smetna, M. Frass, and D. Glogar. Role of beta-endorphins in silent myocardial ischemmia. *Am. J. Cardiol., 58*:428 (1986).

12. G. V. Heller, C. E. Garber, M. J. Connolly, C. F. Allen-Rowlands, S. F. Siconolfi, D. S. Gann, and R. A. Carleton. Plasma beta-endorphin levels in silent myocardial ischemia. *Am. J. Cardiol., 59*:735 (1987).

13. D. S. Sheps, K. F. Adams, A. Hinderliter, C. Price, J. Bissette, G. Orlando, B. Margolis, and G. Koch. Endorphins are related to pain perception in coronary artery disease. *Am. J. Cardiol., 59*:523 (1987).

14. C. Falcone, G. Specchia, R. Rondanelli, L. Guasti, G. Corsico, S. Codega, and C. Montemartini. Correlation between beta-endorphin plasma levels and anginal symptoms in patients with coronary artery disease. *J. Am. Coll. Cardiol., 11*:719 (1988).

3

The Sequence of Events During Episodes of Myocardial Ischemia

Where Does Pain Fit In?

Because of technical and ethical reasons, the direct manipulation of coronary blood flow to induce myocardial ischemia has been difficult to achieve in humans, compared to experimental animal models. Within the past 5 years, however, the advent of percutaneous transluminal coronary angioplasty (PTCA) has provided a unique tool for understanding the sequence of events leading up to the occurrence of pain during episodes of myocardial ischemia in humans. This understanding is an essential component for appreciating the pathophysiology of silent myocardial ischemia. Prior

29

to PTCA, what was known about the sequence of events had been learned from other types of studies. These will be reviewed first.

I. EXERCISE STUDIES

Upton and colleagues [1] used radionuclide ventriculography in 25 coronary artery disease patients and 10 normal controls to evaluate left ventricular dysfunction before angina occurred. These investigators provoked ischemia during two levels of an upright bicycle exercise test. The first radionuclide study during exercise was performed before the onset of ST segment depression and the second one after its appearance. As indicated in Figure 1, the mean ejection fraction increased in the normal subject during the first level of exercise but remained unchanged (an abnormal response) in the patients with coronary artery disease. At the second level of exercise, the control group continued to show an increase, while in the

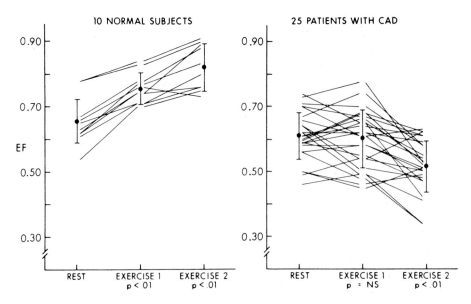

Figure 1   Changes in ejection fraction (EF) from rest to the first level of exercise (exercise 1) and the second level (exercise 2) in 10 normal subjects and 25 patients with coronary artery disease (CAD). (From M. T. Upton, S. K. Rerych, G. E. Newman, S. Port, F. R. Cobb, and R. H. Jones. *Circulation, 62*:341, 1980.)

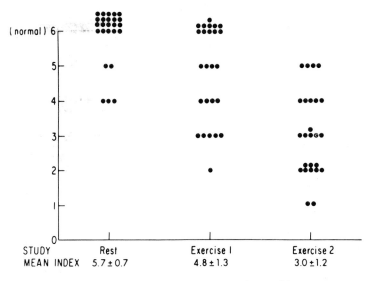

Figure 2   Regional wall motion index in 25 patients with coronary artery disease at rest, exercise 1 and exercise 2. (From M. T. Upton, S. K. Rerych, G. E. Newman, S. Port, F. R. Cobb, and R. H. Jones. *Circulation, 62*:341, 1980. Reproduced with permission of the American Heart Association.)

coronary artery disease group there was now a frank decrease for the group as a whole and all patients showed an abnormal response. Wall motion patterns showed a similar trend (Figure 2). A regional wall motion index was used to assess these changes. At the first level of exercise, 14 of the coronary patients (56%) developed a new wall motion abnormality or demonstrated progression in a preexisting defect at rest. At the second level of exercise, wall motion was abnormal in all patients. Nine of the twenty-five patients with coronary artery disease did not experience angina during these studies. Thus, this study concluded that angina pectoris and ST segment shifts on the electrocardiogram are frequently late manifestations of myocardial ischemia. Another exercise study—this one involving recumbent exercise—showed that regional wall motion changes (determined by echocardiography) began at 30 ± 15 sec after onset of exercise and preceded electrocardiographic changes by an average of 60 sec [2].

II. CONTINUOUS HEMODYNAMIC MONITORING

Possibly the single most important of these studies emanated from Maseri's laboratory. This study by Chierchia et al. [3] is important because of the intensive invasive and noninvasive monitoring that the six patients in the study underwent. These six patients were admitted to the coronary care unit because of transient, recurrent episodes of angina at rest with atypical ST-T changes. To document the location and direction of ST segment changes, 12-lead ECG tracings were recorded in each patient during the course of several angina attacks. In addition to electrocardiographic monitoring, the left ventricular or aortic pressure was continuously monitored, as well as the coronary sinus oxygen saturation. The latter

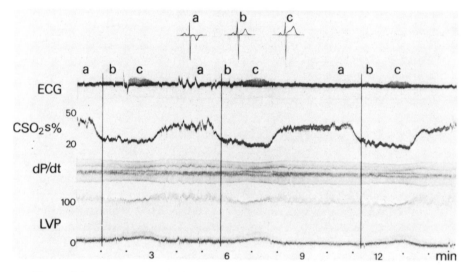

Figure 3 Low-speed playback (paper speed 0.3 mm/sec) of ECG, coronary sinus O_2 saturation (CSO$_2$S), left ventricular pressure (LVP), and dP/dt during three successive asymptomatic episodes recorded over a period of about 15 min. At the top are electrocardiographic patterns (lead V_2) in resting conditions (a), at the onset (b), and at the peak (c) of the ischemic episode. Vertical lines correspond to the onset of the ST-T changes. A sharp drop of CSO$_2$S (denoting reduction in coronary blood flow) consistently precedes the onset of ECG and hemodynamic changes. (From S. Chierchia, I. Simonetti, M. Lazzari, and A. Maseri. *Circulation, 61*:759, 1980. Reproduced with permission of the American Heart Association.)

was assumed to reflect changes in myocardial blood flow, provided the arterial oxygen content and the myocardial oxygen consumption remained constant. Thirty-one episodes of ST segment or T wave abnormalities (most involving ST segment elevation in these mainly Prinzmetal angina patients) were recorded. Only eight episodes were accompanied by typical angina pain.

Although the ischemic episodes were accompanied by different hemo-dynamic patterns in individual patients, some common features were striking. Pain when present occurred 50-120 sec *after* the onset of ST-T wave changes. The authors concluded that pain did not appear to be a reliable and sensitive marker of transient, acute myocardial ischemia. In none of these patients with rest angina were the ST-T changes preceded

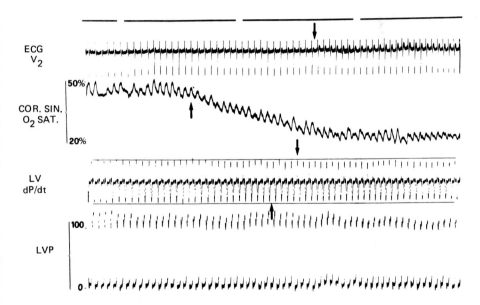

Figure 4   High-speed playback (paper speed 10 mm/sec) of the transient phase of an ischemic episode characterized by peaking of T waves. Arrows indicate the onset of change for each recorded parameter. A drop in CSO_2S (denoting reduction in coronary blood flow) precedes the onset of ECG and hemodynamic changes. (From S. Chierchia, C. Brunelli, I. Simonetti, M. Lazzari, and A. Maseri. *Circulation, 61*:759, 1980. Reproduced with permission of the American Heart Association.)

by consistent increases in the hemodynamic determinants of myocardial oxygen consumption (such as increased heart rate or blood pressure). Hemodynamic changes reflecting acute left ventricular functional impairment did occur before ST changes but even earlier changes than these usually occurred in the coronary sinus oxygen saturation. This presumably reflected decreased myocardial blood flow. Figures 3 and 4 depict the sequence of events: primary reduction in coronary blood flow, fall in left ventricular systolic pressure and left ventricular dP/dt, and a rise in left ventricular end-diastolic pressure, and then ST-T changes. Pain was the final event, when it occurred. The truly ischemic nature of these episodes was confirmed by thallium-201 scintigrams during painless episodes in four patients that showed perfusion defects relative to control tracings. More recently, Levy et al. [4] used ambulatory pulmonary artery monitoring during spontaneous, pacing-induced and exercise-induced ischemia to document a similar sequence. Pain was the final event, occurring after

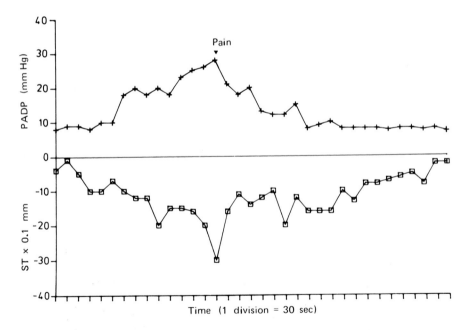

Figure 5 Changes in pulmonary artery diastolic pressure (PADP) and the ST segment during an episode of angina recorded during ambulatory monitoring. (From R. D. Levy, L. M. Shapiro, C. Wright, L. Mockus, and K. M. Fox. *Br. Heart J., 56*:12, 1986.)

the rise in pulmonary artery diastolic pressure and ST segment depression (Figure 5).

III. TRANSIENT CORONARY ARTERY OBSTRUCTION DURING BALLOON ANGIOPLASTY

Sigwart and colleagues [5] were among the first to use this procedure to shed additional light on the sequence of ischemic events. They carefully monitored several variables during balloon obstruction of the coronary arteries in humans. This technique—the key part of the transluminal coronary angioplasty procedure—allows the onset of ischemia to be precisely defined in a controlled setting. In 12 patients, one catheter was placed in the pulmonary artery, and a high-fidelity micromanometer was placed in the left ventricle via the transseptal approach. The time of coronary occlusion was identified by a sudden pressure drop at the distal end of the balloon catheter. Duration of the balloon occlusion was adjusted according to the alteration in the contractility and relaxation variables that were measured. Left ventricular dimensional changes were obtained in five patients with M-mode echocardiography and in five patients with biplane angiography. The time course of various hemodynamic changes is shown in Figure 6. Heart rate and blood pressure changes were small during the first 15 sec of the balloon occlusion (which usually involved the left anterior descending coronary artery), but dP/dt max and dP/dt min (the latter on index of relaxation) fell. Left ventricular end-diastolic pressure changed little. Ejection fraction measured 10 seconds after occlusion in five patients was reduced by over one-third of the control value. Angina, when it occurred, was later than 25 sec after balloon occlusion and was usually preceded by ECG changes.

Figure 7 shows the sequence of events over the course of the first 30 sec after occlusion. It was of interest that the relaxation parameters were the most sensitive of all the variables. This confirmed earlier reports in experimental animals, as well as other studies of transluminal angioplasty in humans. The authors concluded that "ischemia in conscious man is always characterized by a transition period during which it remains silent." As we shall see from other clinical studies in subsequent chapters, the transition to a symptomatic stage does not necessarily occur in many instances of transient myocardial ischemia. Serruys et al. [6] reported similar findings in their studies using cine left ventriculography, but it has been the echocardiogram that has emerged as the prime investigational tool for documenting left ventricular wall motion changes. For example,

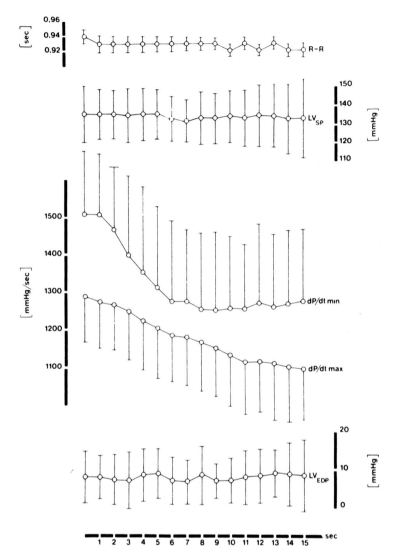

Figure 6 Heart rate (R-R), left ventricular systolic pressure (LV$_{sp}$), dP/dt min, dP/dt max, and left ventricular end-diastolic pressure (LV$_{EDP}$) during the first 15-sec coronary balloon obstruction in 12 patients (mean ± 1 SD). (From U. Sigwart, M. Grbic, M. Payot, J-J. Goy, A. Essinger, and A. Fischer. In *Silent Myocardial Ischemia* [W. Rutishauser and H. Roskamm, eds.], Springer-Verlag, Berlin, 1984.)

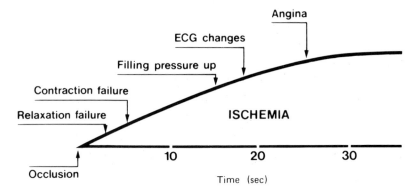

Figure 7 Appearance of events during transient coronary occlusion. (From U. Sigwart, M. Grbic, M. Payot, J-J. Goy, A. Essinger, and A. Fischer. In *Silent Myocardial Ischemia* [W. Rutishauser and H. Roskamm, eds.], Springer-Verlag, Berlin, 1984.)

Hauser et al [7] studied 18 patients with echocardiography during PTCA. Left ventricular wall motion was originally normal in 14. During 22 episodes of angioplasty, hypokinesis, usually rapidly progressing to dyskinesis, occurred 19 ± 8 sec after coronary occlusion. ST segment shifts occurred after 30 ± 5 sec and pain occurred after 39 ± 6 sec (in nine episodes) (Table 1). Similar findings were reported by Visser et al. [8], Alam et al. [9], and Wohlgelernter et al. [10], while Labovitz et al. [11] documented changes in both diastolic and systolic left ventricular function with echocardiographic techniques. The echocardiogram has also been used in other than PTCA studies to define the timing of ischemic events. The experience of Distante and colleagues has been particularly impressive in documenting the "pre-ECG phase" in which left ventricular dysfunction is the only abnormality (Table 2) [12].

IV. CONCLUSIONS

Based on exercise studies, hemodynamic monitoring and most importantly, transient coronary artery obstruction during PTCA, it is clear that pain is the *final* event in the sequence of events that characterizes the ischemic episode. In primary ischemia, there is first a reduction in coronary blood flow followed by hemodynamic evidence of left ventricular

Table 1 Clinical, Electrocardiographic and Echocardiographic Findings in Patients Undergoing Coronary Angioplasty

Case	Age (yr) & sex	Symptoms	PCA vessel (obstruction)	Mean time to dyssynergy (seconds)	Mean time to normalization (sec)	Mean time to ST shift (↑↓) (sec)	Mean time to pain (sec)	Wall motion pre PCA	Wall motion during PCA
1	45M	Stable angina	LAD (95%)	20.5	39	30 ↑	40	Normal	Apical dys.
2	71M	Unstable angina	LAD (80%)	11.5	9	—	52	Mild apical dys.	Marked dys.
3	59M	Postinfarction	LAD (75%)	10	22	30 ↑	30	Mild apical hypo.	Apical dys.
4	60M	Unstable angina	LAD (90%)	22.5	9	—	—	Normal	Apical dys.
5	68F	Unstable angina	RCA (95%)	22.5	20	—	—	Normal	Inferior dys.
6	46M	Unstable angina	LAD (95%)	27.5	15	—	55	Normal	Apical hypo.
			RCA (80%)	22.5	7.5	—	—		Inferior hypo.
7	58M	Stable angina	LAD (90%)	No change	—	—	—	Normal	Normal[a,b]
8	46M	Stable angina	LAD (80%)	32.5	16	40 ↓	45	Normal	Apical dys.[c]
9	63M	Stable angina	LAD (70%)	30	—	—	—	Normal	Apical dys.
			LCx (60%)	No change	—	—	—		Normal[a]
			RCA (90%)	30	—	—	—		Inferior hypo.
10	55M	Stable angina	LAD (90%)	20	80	30 ↑	30	Normal	Apical dys.
11	70F	Unstable angina	LAD (95%)	13.5	15	25 ↓	30	Normal	Apical dys.
12	53M	Unstable angina	LAD (95%)	20	20	—	—	Normal	Apical dys.
13	42M	Stable angina	LAD (90%)	22.5	24.5	—	35	Normal	Apical dys.
14	53F	Unstable angina	LAD (85%)	12	28.5	30 ↓	—	Normal	Apical dys.
			RCA (70%)	25	10	30 ↑	—		Inferior dys.
15	40M	Unstable angina	LAD (75%)	15	12	—	—	Normal	Apical dys.
16	54M	Stable angina	LAD (95%)	No change	—	—	—	Anterior apical akin.	No change
17	60M	Stable angina	RCA (90%)	18	12.5	—	35	Inferior hypo.[d]	Inferior akin.
18	41M	Stable angina	LAD (75%)	13.5	27.5	25 ↓	—	Normal	Apical dys.

[a] Balloon inflations limited to 30 sec duration.
[b] Percutaneous coronary angioplasty vessel highly collateralized.
[c] Mitral valve prolapse normalizes during percutaneous coronary angioplasty (see text).
[d] Normal wall motion after conclusion of percutaneous coronary angioplasty. Akin. = akinesia; dys. = dyskinesia; F = female; hypo. = hypokinesia; LAD = left anterior descending coronary artery; LCx = left circumflex coronary artery; M = male; PCA = percutaneous coronary angioplasty; RCA = right coronary artery; ↑↓ = ST segment elevation or depression, respectively.

Source: A. M. Hauser, V. Gangadharan, R. C. Ramos, S. Gordon and G. C. Timmis, J Am Coll Cardiol, 5:193, 1985.

Table 2 Time Sequence of Echocardiographic Signs During Acute Ischemia with ST-Segment Elevation in Humans (Prinzmetal's Patients)

	Pre-ECG phase	ECG phase	Post-ECG phase
Electrocardiogram	ST =	ST ↑	ST =
Echocardiogram (M-Mode)			
Wall signs			
Motion	↓	↓↓	↑
End-diastolic thickness	↓	↓	=
End-systolic thickness	↓	↓↓	↑
% systolic thickening	↓	↓↓	↑
Cavity signs			
End-diastolic diameter	= /↑	↑	= /↓
End-systolic diameter	↑	↑↑	↓
% fractional shortening	↓	↓↓	↑
Anginal pain	No	Yes/No	No

Abbreviations: ST, no change; ST ↑, ST-segment elevation; ↓, reduction; ↓↓, marked reduction; ↑, increase; ↑↑, marked increased; =, no change; No, absent; Yes, present.
Source: A. Distante. In *Silent Ischemia: Current Concepts and Management* (T. von Arnim, A. Maseri, eds.). Steinkopff, Darmstadt, 1987, p. 98.

dysfunction and then ECG changes. In secondary ischemia, increases in the work of the heart lead to the hemodynamic abnormalities which are followed by ECG changes. Angina—when it occurs—follows the ECG changes.

REFERENCES

1. M. T. Upton, S. K. Rerych, G. E. Newman, S. Port, F. R. Cobb, and R. H. Jones. Detecting abnormalities in left ventricular function during exercise before angina and ST-segment depression. *Circulation, 62*:341 (1980).

2. Y. Sugishita, S. Koseki, M. Matsuda, T. Tamura, I, Yamaguchi, and I. Ito. Dissociation between regional myocardial dysfunction and ECG changes during myocardial ischemia induced by exercise in patients with angina pectoris. *Am. Heart. J., 106*:1 (1983).

3. S. Chierchia, C. Brunelli, I. Simonetti, M. Lazzari, and A. Maseri. Sequence of events in angina at rest: Primary reduction in coronary flow. *Circulation, 61*:759 (1980).

4. R. D. Levy, L. M. Shapiro, C. Wright, L. Mockus, and K. M. Fox. Haemodynamic response to myocardial ischaemia during unrestricted activity, exercise testing, and atrial pacing assessed by ambulatory pulmonary artery pressure monitoring. *Br. Heart J., 56*:12 (1986).

5. U. Sigwart, M. Grbic, M. Payot, J-J. Goy, A. Essinger, and A. Fischer. Ischemic events during coronary artery balloon occlusion. In *Silent Myocardial Ischemia* (W. Rutishauser and H. Roskamm, eds.), Springer-Verlag, Berlin, 1984, pp. 29-36.

6. P. W. Serruys, W. Wijns, M. van Brand, et al. Left ventricular performance, regional blood flow, wall motion and lactate metabolism during transluminal angioplasty. *Circulation, 70*:25 (1984).

7. A. M. Hauser, V. Gangadharan, R. G. Ramos, S. Gordon, and G. C. Timmis. Sequence of mechanical, electrocardiographic and clinical effects of repeated coronary artery occlusion in human beings: Echocardiographic observations during coronary angioplasty. *J. Am. Coll. Cardiol., 5*:193 (1985).

8. C. A. Visser, G. K. David, and G. Kan. Two-dimensional echocardiography during percutaneous transluminal coronary angioplasty. *Am. Heart J., 111*: 1035 (1986).

9. M. Alam, F. Khaja, J. Brymer, M. Marzelli, and S. Goldstein. Echocardiographic evaluation of left ventricular function during coronary artery angioplasty. *Am. J. Cardiol., 57*:20 (1986).

10. D. Wohlgelernter, C. C. Jaffe, H. S. Cabin, L. A. Yeatman, Jr., and M. Cleman. Silent ischemia during coronary occlusion produced by balloon inflation: Relation to regional myocardial dysfunction. *J. Am. Coll. Cardiol., 10*:491 (1987).

11. A. J. Labovitz, M. K. Lewen, M. Kern, M. Vandormael, U. Deligonal, and H. L. Kennedy. Evaluation of left ventricular systolic and diastolic dysfunction during transient myocardial ischemia produced by angioplasty. *J. Am. Coll. Cardiol., 10*:743 (1987).

12. A. Distante. Noninvasive detection of silent myocardial ischemia with echocardiography. In *Silent Ischemia: Current Concepts and Management* (T. von Arnim, A. Maseri, eds.). Steinkopff, Darmstadt, 19878, p. 98.

4

Left Ventricular Dysfunction and Myocardial Blood Flow Disturbances During Episodes of Silent Myocardial Ischemia

Is Less Myocardium at Jeopardy Than During Symptomatic Ischemia?

Altered pain perception by itself is probably not sufficient to explain all episodes of silent myocardial ischemia, as discussed in Chapter 2. For that reason, it has been postulated that in some instances ischemia is "silent" because less myocardium is ischemic compared to that involved in symptomatic episodes. This chapter will review studies that have compared left ventricular function and myocardial blood flow in symptomatic and asymptomatic myocardial ischemia.

The left ventricular studies can be categorized into three major types: (1) hemodynamic changes recorded with catheters in the right and/or left heart chambers, (2) ventriculography performed either invasively with contrast agent, or noninvasively with radionuclide ventriculography, and (3) echocardiography.

I. HEMODYNAMIC CHANGES DURING SILENT MYOCARDIAL ISCHEMIA

One of the most comprehensive of these studies was the report by Chierchia and colleagues [1]. These investigators studied 14 patients admitted to the coronary care unit because of rest angina. Left ventricular (or pulmonary artery) pressures and systemic arterial hemodynamics were measured for a mean of 13.6 hours during continuing electrocardiographic monitoring. Eighty-four percent (or 247) of the 293 episodes of transient ST and segment and T wave changes were completely asymptomatic. Figure 1 shows a computer plot of hemodynamic variables recorded in these episodes. Most (63%) of these asymptomatic episodes were associated with an elevation in the left ventricular end-diastolic or pulmonary artery diastolic pressure of 5 mmHg or more; a smaller number (15%) had elevations of 2-4 mmHg. In 22% there were no changes or less than a 2 mmHg rise in pressure. Peak contraction and relaxation indices using dP/dt (the first derivative of left ventricular pressure) were reduced considerably (to 100 mgHg/sec or more) in over 88% of the asymptomatic episodes. That these hemodynamic changes represented ischemia in these patients was confirmed by primary reductions in coronary sinus blood flow calculated from changes in coronary sinus oxygen saturation. (Although the patients in this series represented examples of coronary vasospasm, not all instances of silent myocardial ischemia are due to this mechanism.)

The hemodynamic changes during the 247 asymptomatic episodes were compared to those occurring during the 46 symptomatic episodes (Figure 2). Comparisons were also made by type of ST segment changes (depression or elevation). It was of interest that the mean duration of the asymptomatic episodes was significantly shorter than the symptomatic episodes (253 $\pm$ 19 sec vs. 674 $\pm$ 396 sec, $p < 0.001$). Furthermore, the left ventricular end-diastolic pressure did not rise as high in the asymptomatic episodes (5.9 $\pm$ 5.0 mmHg vs. 16.5 $\pm$ 6.9 mmHg, $p < 0.001$). Using peak contraction dP/dt as an index of contractility, the authors also reported less of an impairment in systolic function during the asymptomatic

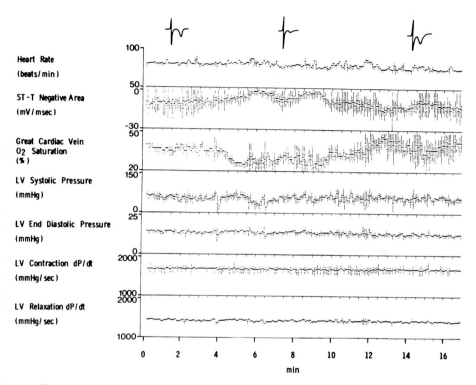

Figure 1 Computer plot of an asymptomatic episode of pseudonormalization of an inverted T wave (decrease in ST-T negative area) in a patient with anterior ischemia. In this patient there was no increase of left ventricular (LV) end-diastolic pressure and the peak contraction and relaxation dP/dt were not altered, although there was a reduction of great cardiac vein oxygen saturation preceding and accompanying the electrocardiographic change. (From S. Chierchia, M. Lazzari, B. Freedman, C. Brunelli, and A. Maseri. *J. Am. Coll. Cardiol.,* *1*:924, 1983.)

episodes (252 ± 156 mmHg/sec vs. 395 ± 199 mmHg/sec, $p < 0.001$). Diastolic function was characterized by peak relaxation dP/dt; again the reduction in this measurement was less in the asymptomatic episodes (259 ± 191 mmHg/sec vs. 413 ± 209 mmHg/sec, $p < 0.001$). These trends were observed regardless of the type of ST segment abnormality. The authors concluded that in their study population, "asymptomatic episodes were usually characterized by a shorter duration and a lesser degree of ischemic left ventricular dysfunction than are the symptomatic episodes, although there is a considerable degree of overlap both in the group data

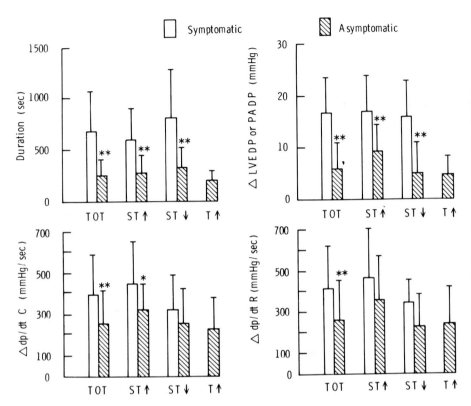

Figure 2 Comparison of symptomatic and asymptomatic episodes of ST segment and T wave changes. The mean values and standard deviation are plotted for the duration of episodes, the increases in left ventricular end-diastolic (LVEDP) (or pulmonary artery diastolic [PADP]) pressure and reductions of left ventricular peak contraction (C) and relaxation (R) dP/dt. P values for comparison of symptomatic and asymptomatic episodes: * = <0.01. ** = <0.001. Overall, asymptomatic episodes were shorter and were accompanied by lesser degrees of left ventricular impairment, ST or = transient ST segment elevation or depression; T = transient pseudonormalizaiton or peaking of inverted or flat T waves; TOT = total. (From S. Chierchia, M. Lazzari, B. Freedman, C. Brunelli, and A. Maseri. *J. Am. Coll. Cardiol., 1*:924, 1983.)

and the results from individual patients.'' The authors speculated that asymptomatic episodes may represent lesser degrees of myocardial ischemia, though they acknowledged that the wide overlap in duration of episodes and degree of left ventricular impairment observed in the group data (as well as multiple episodes in individual patients) indicated that the severity of ischemia was not the only factor involved in the genesis of anginal pain.

II. RADIONUCLIDE AND CONTRAST VENTRICULOGRAPHY

Other investigators have utilized radionuclide ventriculography to evaluate left ventricular function in asymptomatic subjects. Our laboratory [2] employed a computerized program to calculate regional ejection fractions at rest and during exercise. Figure 3 depicts the computer generated left ventricular regions of interest that were evaluated in 40 patients, 16 with and 24 without silent myocardial ischemia. The clinical and arteriographic features of these two groups of patients were similar (Table 1) and so was their ejection fraction response to exercise (Table 2). None of the asymptomatic patients had pain with their test nor were they receiving any antianginal medications that could have modified the pain response. During exercise, global ejection fraction decreased by 0.06 in both groups. Even when differences in resting (baseline) values were considered, the relative decreases were not significant (9% vs. 12%). Analysis of each of the three ventricular regions of interest showed no significant differences in the degree of reduction during exercise. In addition, the percent of normal regions at rest, i.e., with ejection fraction >0.50, that demonstrated a decrease during exercise was 60% in both groups (19/33 vs. 22/46). We concluded that in these 40 patients—in whom the prevalence of myocardial infarction and multivessel disease was similar—no discernible differences in wall motion abnormalities or ejection fraction were present.

Iskandrian and Hakki [3] approached this problem in a slightly different manner. They compared left ventricular function during exercise radionuclide ventriculography in anginal patients who either did or did not have their usual angina during the exercise procedure. Thirty-one patients had angina during the test and 43 did not. Multivessel disease was present in equal percentages in both groups of patients, as were a variety of clinical factors. Although the global ejection fraction was similar at rest in both groups, it fell to a greater extent in the symptomatic group (− 0.045

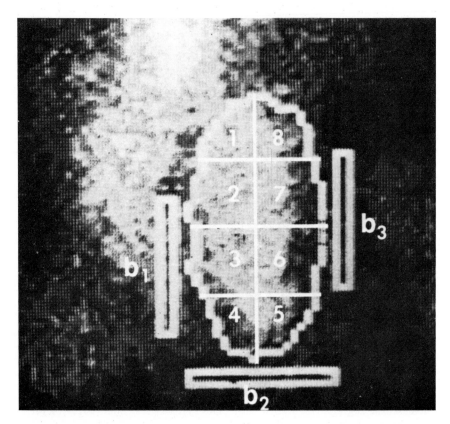

Figure 3   End-diastolic image of heart in left anterior oblique position with hand-drawn left ventricular outline. Eight regions of interest (subdivisions within the left ventricle) are indicated by the numbers 1 to 8. Regions 2 and 3 represent the anteroseptal, 4 and 5 the apical and 6 and 7 the inferoposterior regions. Regions 1 and 8 are not used in analysis of regional ejection fraction because of the overlying cardiac valves and other structures. Three background regions (rectangles b_1, b_2, and b_3 located outside the left ventricular perimeter) are considered using an automated background correction algorithm. (From P. F. Cohn, E. J. Brown, J. Wynne, B. L. Holman, and H. L. Atkins. *J. Am. Coll. Cardiol., 1*:931, 1983.)

Table 1 Clinical and Arteriographic Features in Patients With (Group 1) and Without (Group 2) Silent Myocardial Ischemia

	Group 1 (16 patients)	p	Group 2 (24 patients)
Age (yr)	55 ± 3[a]	NS	54 ± 2
Male	13	NS	19
Prior MI	10	NS	15
CAD			
3 vessel	7	NS	11
2 vessel	6	NS	7
1 vessel	3	NS	6

[a] = mean value ± standard error of the mean.
CAD = coronary artery disease; MI = myocardial infarctions; NS = not significant; p = probability value.
Source: P. F. Cohn, E. J. Brown, J. Wynne, B. L. Holman, and H. L. Atkins. *J. Am. Coll. Cardiol., 1*:931, 1983.

Table 2 Radionuclide Ejection Fraction in Patients With (Group 1) and Without (Group 2) Silent Myocardial Ischemia

	Group 1 (16 patients)	p	Group 2 (24 patients)
Global			
Rest	0.60 ± 0.04	NS	0.53 ± 0.04
Exercise	0.54 ± 0.04	NS	0.47 ± 0.04
Anteroseptal region			
Rest	0.60 ± 0.04	NS	0.51 ± 0.04
Exercise	0.56 ± 0.04	NS	0.45 ± 0.04
Apical region			
Rest	0.65 ± 0.06	NS	0.57 ± 0.05
Exercise	0.62 ± 0.06	NS	0.52 ± 0.05
Inferoposterior region			
Rest	0.70 ± 0.07	NS	0.66 ± 0.05
Exercise	0.64 ± 0.04	NS	0.59 ± 0.05

NS = not significant; p = probability value.
Source: P. F. Cohn, E. J. Brown, J. Wynne, B. L. Holman, and H. L. Atkins. *J. Am. Coll. Cardiol., 1*:931, 1983.

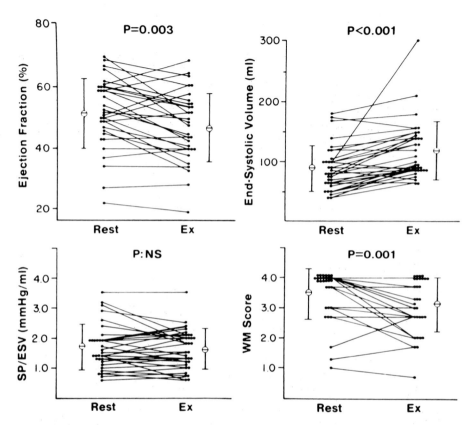

Figure 4   Left ventricular ejection fraction, end-systolic volume, systolic blood pressure-end systolic volume ratio (SP/ESV) and wall motion (WM) score at rest and during exercise (Ex) in patients with angina during the test. The means and standard deviations are also shown. NS = not significant. (From A. S. Iskandrian and A-H. Hakki. *Am. J. Cardiol., 53*:1239, 1984.)

$\pm$ 0.076 vs. -0.01 $\pm$ 0.094, $p < 0.01$). Other measurements (wall motion score, end-systolic volume, etc.) showed similar trends (Figures 4 and 5).

The authors concluded that even though asymptomatic myocardial ischemia may occur in patients with extensive coronary artery disease and be associated with abnormal exercise left ventricular function, in general patients with symptomatic episodes have worse exercise left ventricular function than those with asymptomatic episodes.

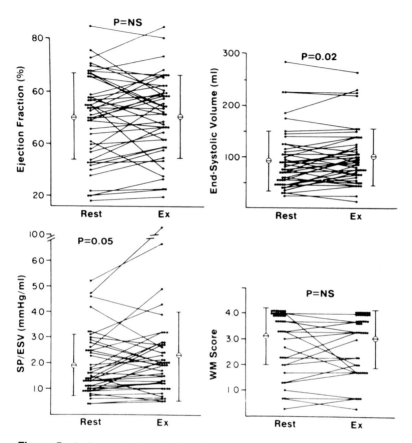

Figure 5 Left ventricular ejection fraction, end-systolic volume, systolic blood pressure-end-systolic volume ratio (SP/ESV) and wall motion (WM) score at rest and during exercise in patients without angina. NS = not significant. (From A. S. Iskandrian and A-H. Hakki. *Am. J. Cardiol.*, 53:1239, 1984.)

Ratib and colleagues [4] performed isotope ventriculography in 25 patients who did not develop chest pain during exercise and found no differences in left ventricular function when compared to 14 patients who did develop angina with exercise (Figure 6). These results are similar to those from our laboratory, as opposed to those of Iskandrian and Hakki. The phase analysis techniques used in this study are different from those of regional ejection fraction analysis, but the results are equally valid.

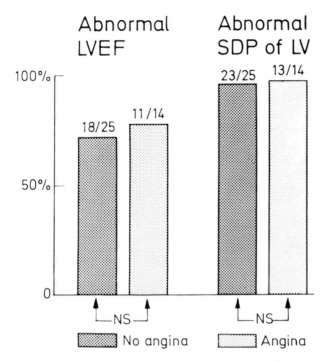

Figure 6 The numbers of patients with an abnormal response of left ventricular (LV) function during exercise. A failure to increase left ventricular ejection fraction (LVEF) by 5% or more was considered abnormal. Using this criterion, 72% of the patients without angina and 78% of the patients with angina had an abnormal LVEF during exercise. The authors established the upper limit of normal for standard deviation of peak (SDP) of LV as 14°, which is the mean plus two standard deviations measured in ten normals at maximum exercise. There was no statistical difference between the two groups. SDP is an index of the degree of synchronicity of LV wall motion. (From O. Ratib, A. Righetti, and W. Rutishauser. In *Silent Myocardial Ischemia* [W. Rutishauser and H. Roskamm, eds.], Springer-Verlag, Berlin, 1984, pp. 84-89.)

Gleichmann and colleagues [5] studied wall motion disorders during contrast ventriculography with bicycle exercise in 141 patients with coronary artery disease. Four combinations were used: angina with wall motion disorders (25% of total group); angina without wall motion disorders (16%); no angina with wall motion disorders (22%); and neither angina nor wall motion disorders (37%). Thus, the presence of angina could not

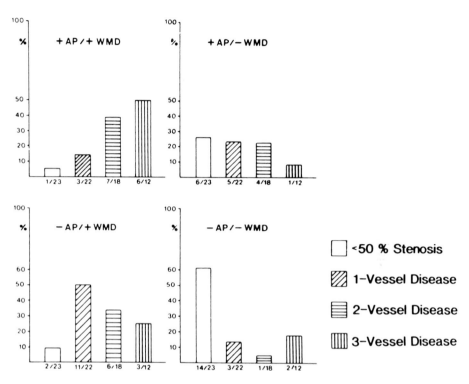

Figure 7 Left ventricular exercise angiography: frequency of angina pectoris (AP) and wall motion disorders (WMD) in 75 patients with coronary artery disease (CAD) without scar. (From U. Gleichmann, D. FaBbender, H. Mannebach, J. Vogt, and G. Trieb. In *Silent Myocardial Ischemia* [W. Rutishauser and H. Roskamm, eds.], Springer-Verlag, Berlin, 1984, pp. 71-77.)

clearly differentiate normal and abnormal left ventricular function with exercise. For example, more than 50% of the patients with one-vessel disease and no prior infarction had no angina but had hypokinesis or akinesis. This combination was less frequent in patients with two-vessel disease (3%) or three-vessel disease (25%). The four possible combinations are depicted in Figure 7. The severe nature of these silent episodes was further confirmed by the rise in left ventricular end-diastolic pressure during exercise in many of the patients with wall motion disorders. However, the higher prevalence of one-vessel disease does suggest less myocardium at jeopardy.

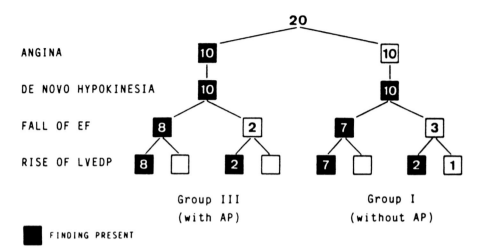

ANGINA

DE NOVO HYPOKINESIA

FALL OF EF

RISE OF LVEDP

Group III
(with AP)

Group I
(without AP)

FINDING PRESENT

Figure 8 Clinical, hemodynamic and angiographic characteristics during exercise in 20 patients with proven coronary artery disease but without prior myocardial infarction. Ten patients were limited by angina, 10 tolerated the exercise test without anginal symptoms. Both patient groups were carefully matched for extent and severity of coronary artery lesions. No differences in prevalence of either regional de novo hypokinesia, decrease of left ventricular ejection fraction (EF) or increase in end-diastolic pressure (LVEDP) were noted between the two groups during exercise at comparable external work loads and rate-pressure products. (From H. O. Hirzel, R. Leutwyler, and H. P. Krayenbuehl. *J. Am. Coll. Cardiol.*, 6:275, 1985.)

Hirzel and colleagues [6] also reported on both wall motion disorders and hemodynamic changes in their series of 36 patients with exercise-induced silent ischemia and 36 matched patients with exercise-induced angina. All patients had a history of angina, but only the latter patients continued to have angina at time of admission, despite the disparity in symptoms. Under similar exercise conditions, comparable hemodynamic and wall motion abnormalities indicative of ischemia were observed in both groups of patients (Figure 8). The authors concluded that "angina pectoris cannot be considered a prerequisite for hemodynamically significant ischemia during exertion." Wall motion abnormalities can also be induced by mental stress. Rozanski and colleagues [7] demonstrated this in 23 of 59 patients with coronary artery disease using radionuclide ventriculography to document the abnormalities, most of which occurred in the absence of symptoms.

A new technique using an ambulatory left ventricular function monitoring device (VEST) has been used to record left ventricular ejection fraction during daily activities. In a recent report, Tamaki et al. (8) reported 36 episodes of transient fall in ejection fraction in 16 angina patients; only 12 were accompanied by typical anginal symptoms. Davies et al. [9] used a precordial scintillation probe to record ventricular volumes in painful and painless ischemia. No significant differences were found.

III. ECHOCARDIOGRAPHY

As noted in Chapter 3, wall motion abnormalities recorded by echocardiography during coronary angioplasty have shown no difference between

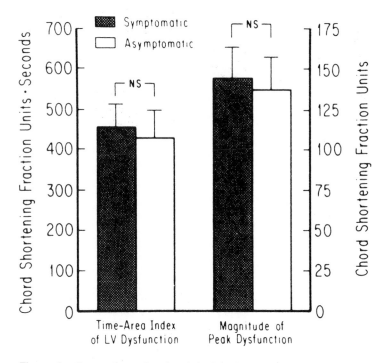

Figure 9 Comparison of regional dysfunction variables in the symptomatic and asymptomatic groups. Brackets represent ±1 SD. There were no differences between the groups in the time-area index of left ventricular (LV) dysfunction or the magnitude of peak dysfunction. (From D. Wohlgelernter, C. C. Jaffe, H. S. Cabin, L. A. Yeatman, Jr., and M. Cleman. *J. Am. Coll. Cardiol., 10*:491, 1987.)

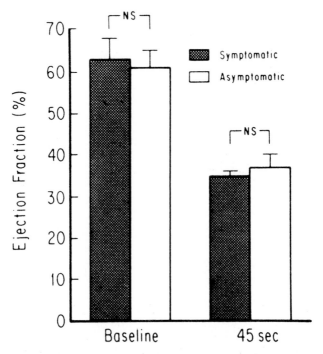

Figure 10 Comparison of global left ventricular ejection fraction responses to balloon inflation in the symptomatic and asymptomatic groups. Brackets represent ±1 SD. There were no differences between the groups in ejection fraction values at baseline or at 45 seconds into inflation. (From D. Wohlgelernter, C. C. Jaffe, H. S. Cabin, L. A. Yeatman, Jr., and M. Cleman. *J. Am. Coll. Cardiol.,* *10*:491, 1987.)

painful and painless episodes. This was most clearly reported by Wohlgelernter et al. [10] in their comparison of regional and global indices of left ventricular dysfunction (Figures 9 and 10), but was also alluded to by others [11].

IV. MYOCARDIAL BLOOD FLOW STUDIES

Myocardial blood flow (perfusion) studies are generally of two types: quantitative (invasive) vs. qualitative (noninvasive). A prime example of the former type is the xenon-133 clearance technique for measuring regional myocardial blood flow. Because of physiologic restraints, this technique has been shown in several centers around the world to be most reliable when the same patient is used as his or her own control. One of the pioneers in this work is Lichtlen. He and his colleagues reported their results in 11 patients with coronary artery disease not experiencing angina during ischemia by rapid atrial pacing [12]. Fifteen patients had angina during these studies and served as a control group. Figure 11 depicts the results: blood flow increased in poststenotic areas much less than in normal regions during rapid atrial pacing, but no differences were found between the angina and nonangina groups. However, individual responses did show a tendency for flow to be actually reduced in some patients with angina (Figure 12). The reason for this is not clear, but a vasospastic mechanism may be implicated.

The prime example of a qualitative, noninvasive method for evaluating myocardial perfusion is the thallium-201 scintigram. Righetti and colleagues [13] found that coronary patients showing perfusion defects without angina had a smaller number of ischemic segments despite a higher double product. By contrast, Reisman et al. [14] found similar amounts of thallium perfusion defects in their patients.

Hinrich and colleagues [15,16] correlated results of lactate extraction and thallium scintigraphy in nine asymptomatic patients with angiographically proven coronary artery disease. In three patients, no myocardial lactate production at rest or after atrial pacing was observed and thallium scintigraphy was normal. Six other patients had both significant defects and lactate production (Figure 13a-c). Coronary sinus blood flow increased to the same degree in both groups of patients. The authors concluded that the absence of metabolic and perfusion abnormalities probably indicated less myocardium at jeopardy, despite the same degree of ST segment depression during atrial pacing or exercise ECG.

Another type of myocardial perfusion technique utilizes an intravenous infusion of rubidium-82. Positron tomograms of rubidium uptake were made for five regions of interest by Deanfield et al. [17] during 24-hour ambulatory monitoring, exercise tests and cold pressor tests in 34 patients with histories of angina. An example of the ECG and perfusion abnormalities with and without angina is depicted in Figure 14. There was no significant difference in the change in uptake of rubidium-82 in the abnormal segment of myocardium between exercise tests accompanied by angina and those without pain (uptake changed from 47 $\pm$ 9.8 to 38 $\pm$ 10.6 for episodes of ST segment depression with angina versus 52 $\pm$ 13 to 44 $\pm$ 12 for episodes of painless ST depression). Similarly, regional uptake changes in the abnormal segment of myocardium during unprovoked

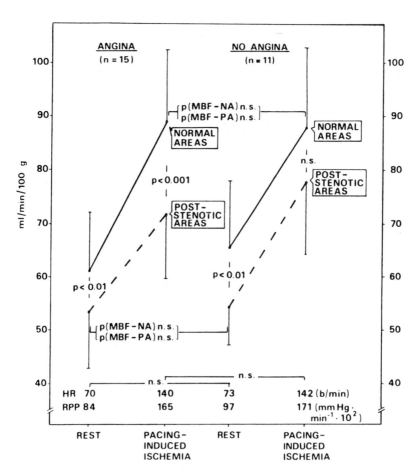

Figure 11 Regional myocardial blood flow (MBF) at rest and during rapid atrial pacing in 15 patients with and 11 patients without angina pectoris during ischemia. NA = normal areas; PA = poststenotic area; HR = heart rate; RPP = rate-pressure product. (From W. G. Daniel, H-J. Engel, H. Hundeshage, and P. R. Lichtlen. In *Silent Myocardial Ischemia* [W. Rutishauser and H. Roskamm, eds.], Springer-Verlag, Berlin, 1984, pp. 45-49.)

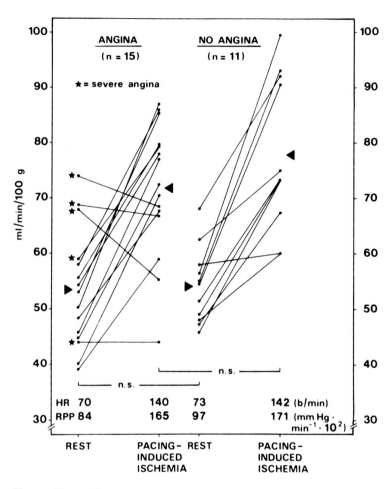

Figure 12 Regional myocardial blood flow in poststenotic areas of 15 patients with and 11 patients without angina pectoris during rapid atrial pacing-induced ischemia. * = severe angina. (From W. G. Daniel, H-J. Engel, H. Hundeshage, and P. R. Lichtlen. In *Silent Myocardial Ischemia* [W. Rutishauser and H. Roskamm, eds.], Springer-Verlag, Berlin, pp. 45-49.)

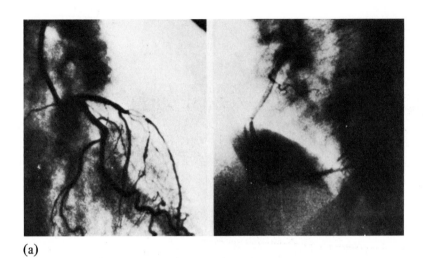

(a)

(b)

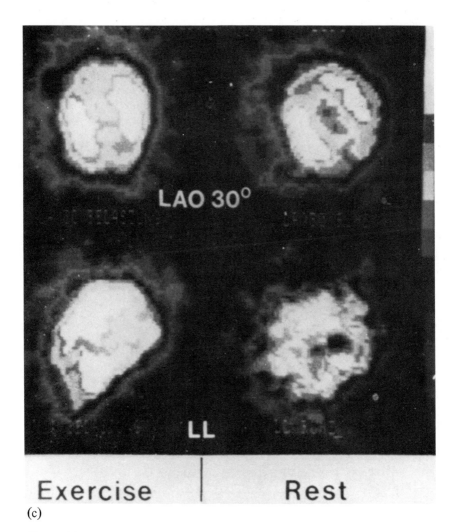

(c)

Exercise | Rest

Figure 13a-c Asymptomatic patient with severe left anterior descending (LAD) stenoses (a) corresponding to ST-segment depression and myocardial lactate production (b), and a reversible thallium defect of the left ventricular anterior wall (c) during exercise or atrial pacing. LAO = left anterior oblique view; LL = left lateral view. (From A. Hinrichs, W. Kupper, C. L. V. Hamm, and W. Bleifeld. In *Silent Myocardial Ischemia* [W. Rutishauser and H. Roskamm, eds.], Springer-Verlag, Berlin, 1984, pp. 50-57.)

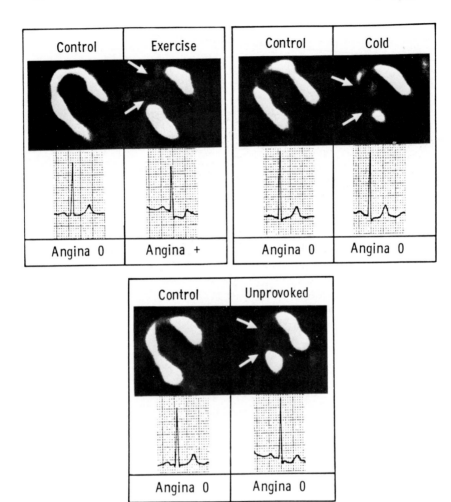

Figure 14 The tomographic slices for a single patient through the midleft ventricle showing the regional myocardial uptake of rubidium-82 in the posterior wall (PW), free wall (FW), anterior wall (a) and interventricular septum (S_1 and S_2) of the left ventricle. This demonstrates the distribution of regional perfusion during control, cold pressor, unprovoked ST depression and exercise. Evidence of regional ischemia occurred during all three tests and supported the ST segment changes as evidence of ischemia whether or not chest pain occurred. (From J. E. Deanfield, P. Ribiero, K. Oakley, S. Krikler, and A. P. Selwyn. *Am. J. Cardiol., 54*: 1195, 1984.)

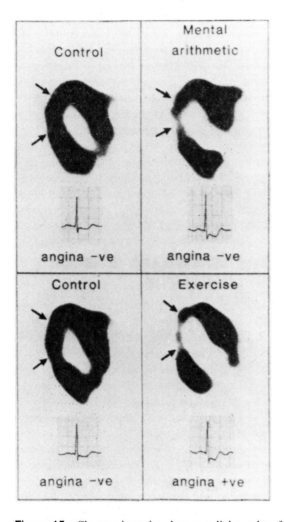

Figure 15 Changes in regional myocardial uptake of ribudium-82, and in ECG in relation to chest pain before and after mental arithmetic or exercise. Control scans show homogeneous regional cation uptake. Patient No. 9 shows anterior and free-wall ischaemia and ST-segment depression with mental arithmetic and exercise, but angina only after exercise (− ve = negative; + ve = positive). (From J. E. Deanfield, M. Kensett, R. A. Wilson, M. Shea, P. Horlock, C. M. deLandsheere, and A. P. Selwyn. *Lancet, 2*:1001, 1984.)

episodes of ST depression with angina were not significantly different from those found during painless episodes (from 48 ± 8.5 to 36 ± 6.6 for episodes of ST segment depression with angina versus 48 ± 7 to 37.5 ± 8.3 for episodes of painless ST depression). The same investigative group has also documented impressive perfusion abnormalities when silent myocardial ischemia occurred during mental arithmetic [18] (Figure 15) and smoking [19]. These studies tend to refute the hypothesis that lesser amounts of myocardium are injured during painless ischemia. The same conclusions can be inferred from the coronary angioplasty studies cited earlier, even though myocardial blood flow was not measured in these studies. At similar durations of occlusion and at similar occlusion pressures (with presumably similar degrees of reduction in myocardial blood flow) there were no differences in degree of left ventricular dysfunction or other indices of myocardial performances.

V. SILENT MYOCARDIAL ISCHEMIA AND "STUNNED" OR "HIBERNATING" MYOCARDIUM

The terms "stunned" [20] or "hibernating" myocardium [21] have been used to describe respectively (1) a state of prolonged postischemic myocardial dysfunction following severe transient ischemia, and (2) reduced myocardial inotropy due to a persistent state of reduced coronary blood flow, i.e., chronic ischemia. It is thought that the reduced inotropy in the latter state may be a protective mechanism whereby the reduced oxygen demand secondary to the reduced inotropy minimizes the extent of ischemia, necrosis, or both [22]. That the myocardium in both postulated states is not irreversibly damaged is suggested by a series of studies documenting contractile reserve (after appropriate stimuli) in coronary patients with depressed left ventricular function [22,23]. The clinical relevance of these syndromes, especially "stunning," is further demonstrated by exercise studies in which hemodynamic and metabolic evidence of ischemia presents long after the symptoms and ECG findings have disappeared [23]. How can silent ischemia contribute to this picture and what are the clinical implications? If patients are unaware of the ischemic episodes that lead to stunned or hibernating myocardium, they may not take the necessary antiischemic agents that can reverse the hemodynamic and metabolic abnormalities. Thus, multiple episodes of silent ischemia may lead to a chronic ischemic state marked by persistent left ventricular dysfunction, and perhaps even electrical instability. Whether an actual ischemic cardiomyopathy—with pathological changes as well—can result is still unclear, but reported cases of ischemic cardiomyopathy presenting de noveau without prior angina or infarction suggests this is possible.

VI. CONCLUSIONS

The majority of studies evaluating hemodynamic, ventriculographic, and myocardial blood flow changes during silent myocardial ischemia do not show any clearcut evidence that less myocardium is at jeopardy during painless episodes compared to symptomatic episodes. Whether these painless ischemic changes can account for some of the left ventricular dysfunction observed in "stunned" or "hibernating" myocardium is an intriguing concept. If so, "chronic" ischemia may be a real entity after all.

REFERENCES

1. S. Chierchia, M. Lazzari, B. Freedman, C. Brunelli, and A. Maseri. Impairment of myocardial perfusion and function during painless myocardial ischemia. *J. Am. Coll. Cardiol., 1*:924 (1983).

2. P. F. Cohn, E. J. Brown, J. Wynne, B. L. Holman, and H. L. Atkins. Global and regional left ventricular ejection fraction abnormalities during exercise in patients with silent myocardial ischemia. *J. Am. Coll. Cardiol., 1*:931 (1983).

3. A. S. Iskandrian and A-H. Hakki. Left ventricular function in patients with coronary heart disease in the presence or absence of angina pectoris during exercise radionuclide ventriculography. *Am. J. Cardiol., 53*:1239 (1984).

4. O. Ratib, A. Righetti, and W. Rutishauser. Isotope ventriculography during asymptomatic ischemia. In *Silent Myocardial Ischemia* (W. Rutishauser and H. Roskamm, eds.), Springer-Verlag, Berlin, 1984, pp. 84-89.

5. D. FaBbender, J. Vogt, H. Mannebach, and U. Gleichmann. Regional wall motion disorders during exercise with and without angina. In *Silent Ischemia: Current Concepts and Management* (T. von Arnim, A. Maseri, eds.). Steinkopff, Darmstadt, 1987, p. 88.

6. H. O. Hirzel, R. Leutwyler, and H. P. Krayenbuehl. Silent myocardial ischemia: Hemodynamic changes during dynamic exercise in patients with proven coronary artery disease despite absence of angina pectoris. *J. Am. Coll. Cardiol., 6*:275, 1985.

7. A. Rozanski, C. N. Biarey, D. S. Krantz, J. Friedman, K. J. Resser, M. Morell, S. Hilton-Chalfen, L. Hestrin, J. Bietendorf, and D. S. Berman. Mental stress and the induction of silent myocardial ischemia in patients with coronary artery disease. *N. Engl. J. Med., 318*:1005 (1988).

8. N. Tamaki, T. Yasuda, R. H. Moore, J. B. Gill, C. A. Boucher, A. H. Hutter Jr., H. G. Gold, and H. W. Strauss. Continuous monitoring of left ventricular

function by an ambulatory radionuclide detector in patients with coronary artery disease. *J. Am. Coll. Cardiol., 12*:669 (1988).

9. G. J. Davies, W. Bencivelli, G. Fragasso, S. Chierchia, F. Crea, J. Crow, P. A. Crean, T. Pratt, M. Morgan, and A. Maseri. Sequence and magnitude of ventricular volume changes in painful and painless myocardial ischemia. *Circulation, 78*:310 (1988).

10. D. Wohlgelernter, C. C. Jaffee, H. S. Cabin, L. A. Yeatman, Jr., and M. Cleman. Silent ischemia during coronary occlusion produced by balloon inflation: Relation to regional myocardial dysfunction. *J. Am. Coll. Cardiol., 10*:491 (1987).

11. A. M. Hauser, V. Gangadhran, R. G. Ramos, S. Gordon, and G. C. Timmis. Sequence of mechanical, electrocardiographic and clinical effects of repeated coronary artery occlusion in human beings: Echocardiographic observations during coronary angioplasty. *J. Am. Coll. Cardiol., 5*:193 (1985).

12. W. G. Faniel, H-J. Engel, H. Hundeshage, and P. R. Lichtlen. Regional myocardial blood flow under rapid atrial pacing in patients with ST-segment depression without angina pain. In *Silent Myocardial Ischemia* (W. Rutishauser and H. Roskamm, eds.), Springer-Verlag, Berlin, 1984, pp. 45-49.

13. A. Righetti, O. Ratib, B. El-Harake, and W. Rutishauser. Thallium-201 myocardial scintigraphy and electrographic findings in asymptomatic coronary patients during exercise testing. In *Silent Myocardial Ischemia* (W. Rutishauser and H. Roskamm, eds.), Springer-Verlag, Berlin, 1984, pp. 79-83.

14. S. Reisman, D. S. Berman, J. Maddahi, and H. J. C. Swan. Silent myocardial ischemia during treadmill exercise. Thallium scintigraphic and angiographic correlates (abstr). *J. Am. Coll. Cardiol., 5*:406 (1985).

15. A. Hinrichs, W. Kupper, C. L. V. Hamm, and W. Bleifeld. Detection of silent myocardial ischemia in correlation to hemodynamic and metabolic data. In *Silent Myocardial Ischemia* (W. Rutihauser and H. Roskamm, eds.), Springer-Verlag, Berlin, 1984, pp. 50-57.

16. C. W. Hamm, W. Kupper, A. Hinrichs, and W. Bleifeld. Identification of patients with silent myocardial ischemia by metabolic, scintigraphic and angiographic findings. In *Silent Ischemia: Current Concepts and Management* (T. von Arnim, A. Maseri, eds.). Steinkopff, Darmstadt, 1987, p. 72.

17. J. E. Deanfield, M. Shea, P. Ribiero, C. M. deLandsheere, R. A. Wilson, P. Horlock, and A. P. Selwyn. Transient ST segment depression as a marker of myocardial ischemia during daily life: A physiological validation in patients with angina and coronary disease. *Am. J. Cardiol., 54*:1195 (1984).

18. J. E. Deanfield, M. Kensett, R. A. Wilson, M. Shea, P. Horlock, C. M. deLandsheere, and A. P. Selwyn. Silent myocardial ischemia due to mental stress. *Lancet, 2*:1001 (1984).

19. J. E. Deanfield, M. T. Shea, R. Wilson, C. M. deLandsheere, A. Jonathan, and A. P. Selwyn. Direct effect of smoking on the heart: Silent ischemic disturbances of coronary flow. *Am. J. Cardiol., 57*:1005 (1986).

20. E. Braunwald and R. A. Kloner. The stunned myocardium: prolonged, postischemic ventricular dysfunction. *Circulation, 66*:1146 (1982).

21. E. Braunwald and J. D. Rutherford. Reversible ischemic left ventricular dysfunction: evidence for the hibernating myocardium. *J. Am. Coll. Cardiol., 8*:1467 (1986).

22. A. S. Iskandrian, J. Heo, R. H. Helfant, and B. L. Segal. Chronic myocardial ischemia and left ventricular function. *Ann. Intern. Med., 107*:925 (1987).

23. B. Patel, R. A. Kloner, K. Przyklenk, and E. Braunwald. Postischemic myocardial "stunning": A clinically relevant phenomenon. *Ann. Intern. Med., 108*:626 (1988).

II

PREVALENCE OF ASYMPTOMATIC CORONARY ARTERY DISEASE

5
Prevalence of Silent Myocardial Ischemia

The actual number of persons with silent myocardial ischemia is not yet known, but intelligent estimates are possible based on data available in the medical literature. These data suggest that the presence of pain in persons with coronary artery disease is just the "tip of the iceberg"; i.e., many individuals are free of pain during most ischemic episodes. Some never have pain.

I. SILENT MYOCARDIAL ISCHEMIA IN PERSONS WITH TOTALLY ASYMPTOMATIC CORONARY ARTERY DISEASE

This is the most difficult area to obtain "hard data" in. How are persons who are free of symptoms to be convinced of the need to undergo coronary arteriography in order to confirm the diagnosis of asymptomatic coronary artery disease? It is true that fortuitous—and anecdotal—"case finding" in this syndrome occurs commonly enough to draw attention to the problem, but systematic surveys are rare. This is because of concerns raised about subjecting asymptomatic individuals to an invasive procedure with a small but definite morbidity and mortality. For example, mortality as a result of cardiac catheterization and angiography can range from 0 to 1% in different centers.

Another approach to estimating the prevalence of asymptomatic disease is through pathologic surveys of atherosclerotic heart disease in adult populations who were apparently free of clinical coronary artery disease at time of death, and died of trauma or noncardiac causes. Diamond and Forrester conducted a comprehensive review in 1979 [1]. They summarized their data in Table 1, which breaks down the autopsy studies by age and sex. In the nearly 24,000 persons studied, the mean prevalence of coronary artery disease was 4.5%. The population-weighted mean (obtained by use of the 1970 U.S. Census figures) was 6.4 ± 0.2% for men

Table 1 Prevalence of Coronary Artery Stenosis at Autopsy

	Men		Women	
Age (yr)	Proportion affected	Pooled mean ± SEP[a] (%)	Proportion affected	Pooled mean ± SEP (%)
30-39	57/2,954	1.9 ± 0.3	5/1,545	0.3 ± 0.1
40-49	234/4,407	5.5 ± 0.3	18/1,778	1.0 ± 0.2
50-59	488/5,011	9.7 ± 0.4	62/1,934	3.2 ± 0.4
60-69	569/4,641	12.3 ± 0.5	130/1,726	7.5 ± 0.6
Totals	1,348/17,013		215/6,983	
Population-weighted mean[b]		6.4 ± 0.2		2.6 ± 0.2

[a]Standard error of the per cent.
[b]Population weighting was performed by use of the 1970 U.S. Census figures.
Source: G. A. Diamond and J. S. Forrester. *N. Engl. J. Med., 300*:1350, 1979.

aged 30-69 and 2.6 ± 0.2% for women aged 30-69. This percentage increased with increasing age. Since these figures are obtained from autopsy data, they may overestimate the true incidence of this syndrome for two reasons. First, unless the autopsy procedure employs techniques for injecting the coronary arteries, the "collapsed" lumen examined by the pathologist may exaggerate the luminal narrowing caused by a given lesion during life. Second, even when the degree of narrowing is as it was during life, there is no certainty that lesions in the 50-60% category were hemodynamically significant when the person was alive. In other words, not all asymptomatic coronary artery disease present at autopsy is necessarily ischemia-producing coronary artery disease. Just as those lesions were not hemodynamically significant, others may represent "end-stage" or "burned-out" stages of the disease process: arteries became occluded, infarctions occurred, scar tissue formed, but there is no longer evidence of active ischemia.

Another approach to estimating the prevalence of coronary artery disease in asymptomatic persons is by reviewing coronary angiographic data. In their report, Diamond and Forrester [1] also performed that type of analysis. Their data suggested that the prevalence of coronary artery disease in asymptomatic adults was about 4%. These patients had undergone cardiac catheterization for reasons other than chest pain (evaluation of valvular heart disease, abnormal ECGs, etc.). Since these catheterization laboratory figures reflect a skewered population in that they were selected to undergo the procedure, one might argue that the 4% figure is too low. Perhaps an "average" of the autopsy and angiographic figures (about 5%) would be more useful. However, in neither the autopsy review nor the angiographic review are data supplied about the prevalence of active ischemia in these asymptomatic subjects.

Screening large numbers of asymptomatic persons with exercise tests and *then* subjecting positive responders to coronary angiography is a useful technique for estimating the number of individuals with *both* asymptomatic disease and active ischemia. Several such studies have been reported. In one small study, investigators at Yale University [2] exercised 129 workers in a nearby industrial plant. Sixteen subjects had an abnormal exercise test and 13 of these also had coronary artery calcification on fluoroscopy. The 13 men underwent coronary arteriography; 12 had at least 50% stenosis in one coronary artery. Thus, 12 of the anginal 129 subjects, or about 9%, had both symptomatic coronary artery disease and silent myocardial ischemia. U.S. Air Force studies in 1390 men revealed 111 with positive exercise tests in a single lead, of which 34 (or about

2.5%) had lesions of at least 50% stenosis [3]. The mean age of these patients was 43 years; all were males. In Norway, Erikssen and Thaulow [4] studied 2014 male office workers who were aged 40-59 years (mean age 50). Sixty-nine had at least 50% stenosis in one coronary artery and 50 of these (or 2.8% of the total) were completely asymptomatic. This percentage is very similar to that in the U.S. Air Force study.

These figures must be considered as conservative estimates, since it is possible that some asymptomatic individuals did not manifest silent ischemia on the one screening exercise test and, therefore, were not selected for coronary angiographic studies. Furthermore, exercise tests in general have a certain percentage of false-negative tests, whereas coronary angiography tends to underestimate the severity of lesions. Thus, the figure of 5% cited earlier for the prevalence of asymptomatic anatomic disease probably exaggerates only slightly the true prevalence of hemodynamically significant asymptomatic disease i.e., disease capable of producing ischemia during physiologic stress. If one assumes that 4% of asymptomatic middle-aged males in the United States have silent myocardial ischemia, then we are considering a total of nearly two million men, not an insignificant sum.

II. SILENT MYOCARDIAL ISCHEMIA IN INDIVIDUALS ASYMPTOMATIC AFTER A MYOCARDIAL INFARCTION

It has been estimated that about 500,000 hospitalized patients survive myocardial infarctions annually in the United States. Of these, 30-40% have their courses complicated by persistent angina, heart failure or serious arrhythmias. The rest are asymptomatic at time of discharge. Of these 300,000 or so individuals, about one-third (100,000) have evidence of ischemia on postinfarction exercise tests. The proportion that are pain free on their tests differs from study to study, ranging from one-third to two-thirds [5-8]. Thus, based on exercise test data, about 50,000 asymptomatic postinfarction patients per year have silent myocardial ischemia in the initial 30-day postinfarction period. In patients who are unable to exercise, Holter monitoring has been used to document the occurrence of silent ischemia [9].

III. SILENT MYOCARDIAL ISCHEMIA IN PATIENTS WITH ANGINA

The number of patients with angina who also have symptomatic episodes of myocardial ischemia is large, but the exact percentage is unknown.

Table 2 Myocardial Ischemia Without Anginal Symptoms

| | Patients with CAD manifesting abnormality | | |
| | | Group with angina[a] | |
Abnormality suggestive of myocardial ischemia	Total group (n)	no.	%
Abnormal left ventricular wall motion	87	33	39%
Pacing contrast ventriculogram[1]	8	3	38%
Pacing contrast ventriculogram[2]	8	6	75%
Exercise radionuclide ventriculogram[5]	63	18	29%
Exercise radionuclide ventriculogram[6]	8	6	75%
Abnormal lactate metabolism	36	9	25%
Pacing study[7]	14	1	7%
Pacing study[8]	22	8	36%
Abnormal myocardial perfusion scintigrams	64	26	40%
Thallium-201 study[9]	35	20	57%
Rubidium-81 study[10]	29	6	19%
Electrocardiographic stress test	568	186	32%
Treadmill test[11]	135	23	17%
Treadmill test[12]	122	32	26%
Bicycle and two-step test[13]	59	15	26%
Treadmill test[14]	146	68	45%
Treadmill test[15]	102	48	47%
Total	755	254	34%

[a]Although not symptomatic during this test, almost all patients in these studies had a history of angina or prior myocardial infarction (see text).
CAD = coronary artery disease.
Source: P. F. Cohn. *Am. J. Cardiol.*, 45:697, 1980. (Numbers in superscript refer to studies cited in this article.)

About 3-4 million patients per year in the United States are seen by physicians because of anginal complaints. When I initially reviewed the literature on positive exercise tests, lactate determinations, abnormal ventriculograms, etc. in those studies that reported symptoms, I found that about a third of asymptomatic patients (Table 2) had at least one documented episode of silent myocardial ischemia [10]. The widespread use of Holter monitoring in the angina population has provided additional data [11-14]. In general, about half of the patients with angina (stable or unstable) have silent ischemia on Holter monitoring, with some series reporting much higher frequencies in their study population [15]. In apparently adequately treated patients, the figure drops to about one-third [16]. Furthermore,

(a) 10:53 A.M. MODIFIED V1 (Shortly after Leaving Clinic)

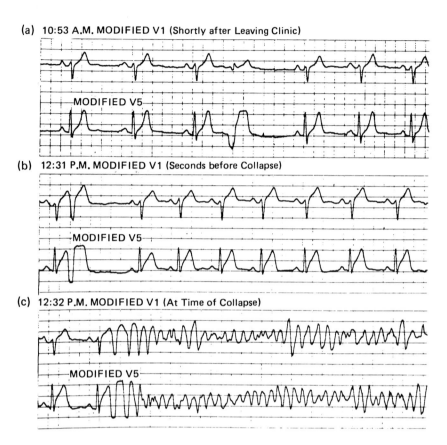

(b) 12:31 P.M. MODIFIED V1 (Seconds before Collapse)

(c) 12:32 P.M. MODIFIED V1 (At Time of Collapse)

Figure 1 (a) The subject's first ventricular premature depolarization, which was detected approximately a half hour after he left the clinic. No significant changes in the S-T segment were noted at the time of this late-cycle premature depolarization. (b) The second form of ventricular premature depolarization, which was uniformly early-cycle and associated with increased S-T segment elevation and convex S-T segment morphology. (c) The electrocardiogram at the instant of the subject's collapse. The same early-cycle ventricular premature form detected earlier initiated a four-beat run of ventricular tachycardia, which rapidly degenerated to ventricular flutter-fibrillation. (From D. D. Savage, W. P. Castelli, S. J. Anderson, and W. B. Kannel. *Am. J. Med., 74*:148, 1983.)

the silent episodes outnumber the painful ones at least three or four to one in both conditions. This is discussed in Chapter 8.

IV. SUDDEN DEATH AND MYOCARDIAL INFARCTION IN PATIENTS WITHOUT PRIOR HISTORIES OF ANGINA

Although this is an "indirect" way of estimating the population with asymptomatic coronary artery disease, it provides important data. Presumably, individuals who die suddenly or experience a myocardial infarction as their initial manifestation of coronary artery disease and who have extensive coronary atherosclerosis at autopsy or coronary angiography did not develop those lesions overnight. Much of the disease must have been present, silent and undetected, for weeks, months, or even years prior to the actual event. This is the natural history—amply documented—of coronary atherosclerosis. That the precipitating event, such as rupture of a plaque into a vessel lumen, could have been sudden is not in dispute, but the atherosclerotic substrate took months and years to develop. With that in mind, it is important to note that in most series one-quarter to one-half of the individuals who die suddenly each year with coronary artery disease found at autopsy had no prior cardiac history [17-19], though some series report a smaller percentage [20]. It is estimated that between 250,000 and 350,000 deaths/year are sudden; therefore, the number of persons without overt coronary artery disease is large by any standard.

Table 3 Catheterization Data in Myocardial Infarction Patients

Parameter	Group 1: No prior AP	Group 2: AP prior to MI	Sig
Mean EDP (mmHg)	15.8 ± 6.9	14.5 ± 6.5	NS
Mean LVEF (%)	58.7 ± 14.7	58.5 ± 14.8	NS
Collaterals	46%	71%	$p < 0.05$
One-vessel disease	38/63 (60%)	3/34 (9%)	$p < 0.005$
Two-vessel disease	18/63 (29%)	18/34 (53%)	$p < 0.05$
Three-vessel disease	7/63 (11%)	13/34 (38%)	$p < 0.005$

Abbreviations: AP, angina pectoris; Sig, significance; MI, myocardial infarction; EDP, end-diastolic pressure; LVEF, left ventricular ejection fraction; NS, not significant.
Source: J. Midwall, J. Ambrose, A. Pichard, Z. Abedin, and M. V. Herman. *Chest, 81*:6, 1982.

As Kuller [18] has written, "The large pool of individuals currently over the age of 30 or 40 with silent but significant coronary atherosclerosis and stenoses will contribute to a high incidence of sudden death, at least for the next 20 or 30 years." Savage et al. [21] provide a graphic example of death in one such individual recorded on an ambulatory monitor that was performed fortuitously as part of a Framingham study protocol (Figure 1).

Nearly half of the patients presenting with their first myocardial infarctions have not had angina beforehand [22-27]. Midwall and colleagues [23] noted that in general, these patients were more likely to be younger, female, and have a greater prevalence of one-vessel disease (Table 3). Pierard et al. [24] reported a 39% prevalence in a series of 732 consecutive patients. Patients without preceeding angina were younger, more likely to be men, and had a higher frequency of inferior infarction and lower frequency of postinfarction angina (Table 4). Matsuda et al. [25] reported a lower ejection fraction in patients without antecedent angina, even when coronary anatomy was similar. The same investigators also showed an almost equal likelihood of the infarction occurring at rest as with exertion [26]. In a report from our hospital [27], we studied 43 consecutive patients presenting with their initial myocardial infarction; 23 had no history of angina prior to the infarction, whereas 20 did. The two groups did not differ in age, smoking history, diabetes, hypertension, or cholesterol levels. The prevalence of Q and non-Q wave infarcts was similar, but there was a trend toward more inferior infarctions in the asymptomatic group (65% vs. 47%) and more single-vessel disease (40% vs. 11%). Multivessel coronary artery disease is frequent enough, however, in patients without prior angina to suggest that an infarction without prior angina does not necessarily indicate less advanced coronary artery disease and, therefore, should not be considered a unique subset of coronary artery disease.

V. CONCLUSIONS

Silent myocardial ischemia is a ubiquitous phenomenon, present in almost 5% of the asymptomatic population, about one-third of uncomplicated asymptomatic postinfarction patients and in many patients with angina. The scope of the problem is further indicated—albeit indirectly—by the large number of individuals dying suddenly or experiencing an infarction without a prior anginal history.

Table 4 Comparison Between Patients With or Without Angina Pectoris Before Infarction

	Patients with angina before infarction	Patients without angina before infarction	p value
Pts (n)	447	285	
Time interval between onset of pain and admission (hours)	13 ± 24	10 ± 16	<0.05
Mean age (yr)	59 ± 9	57 ± 11	<0.05
Sex (% women)	22	12	<0.001
Prior history of diabetes mellitus (%)	11	8	NS
Tobacco abuse (%)	80	86	<0.05
Medications before infarction			
Beta blockers (%)	15	3	<0.001
Diuretics (%)	12	7	<0.05
Digitalis (%)	5	4	NS
Antiarrhythmics (%)	3	1	<0.05
Site of infarction			
Non-Q-wave (%)	11	11	NS
Anterior (%)	43	33	<0.01
Inferior (%)	44	55	<0.01
Unknown (%)	2	1	NS
Peak creatine kinase (IU/liter)	1,454 ± 1,142	1,569 ± 1,099	NS
Worst LV function score during hospital stay	1.0 ± 1.2	1.0 ± 1.1	NS
Early post-infarction angina (%)	21	10	<0.001
In-hospital recurrent infarction (%)	2	1	NS
Pericardial friction rub (%)	26	25	NS
Bradycardia (%)	17	17	NS
Atrial fibrillation (%)	16	11	NS
Frequent PVCs (%)	42	44	NS
Ventricular tachycardia (%)	6	5	NS
Ventricular fibrillation (%)	9	9	NS
Atrioventricular block (%)	11	15	NS
Bundle branch block (%)	9	10	NS
In-hospital mortality (%)	10	8	NS
3-year post-hospital mortality (%)	16	7	<0.001

LV = left ventricular; NS = difference not significant; PVCs = premature ventricular complexes.
Source: L. A. Pierard, C. Dubois, J-P. Smeets, J. Boland, J. Carlier, and H. E. Kulbertus. *Am. J. Cardiol., 61*:984, 1988.

REFERENCES

1. G. A. Diamond and J. S. Forrester. Analysis of probability as an aid in the clinical diagnosis of coronary artery disease. *N. Engl. J. Med., 300*:1350 (1979).

2. R. A. Langou, E. K. Huang, M. J. Kelley, and L. S. Cohen. Predictive accuracy of coronary artery calcification and abnormal exercise test for coronary artery disease in asymptomatic men. *Circulation, 62*:1196 (1980).

3. V. F. Froelicher, A. J. Thompson, M. R. Longo, Jr., J. H. Triebwasser, and M. C. Lancaster. Value of exercise testing for screening symptomatic men for latent coronary artery disease. *Prog. Cardiolvasc. Dis., 16*:265 (1976).

4. J. Erikssen and E. Thaulow. Follow-up of patients with asymptomatic myocardial ischemia. In *Silent Myocardial Ischemia* (W. Rutishauser, H. Roskamm, eds.). Springer-Verlag, Berlin, 1984, pp. 156-164.

5. P. Theroux, D. D. Waters, C. Halphen, J-C. Debaisieux, and H. F. Mizgala. Prognostic value of exercise testing soon after myocardial infarction. *N. Engl. J. Med., 301*:341 (1979).

6. D. H. Miller and J. D. Borer. Exercise testing early after myocardial infarction: risks and benefits. *Am. J. Med., 72*:427 (1982).

7. D. A. Weiner, R. J. Ryan, C. H. McCabe, S. Luk, B. R. Chaitman, L. T. Sheffield, F. Tristani, and L. D. Fisher. Significance of silent myocardial ischemia during exercise testing in patients with coronary artery disease. *Am. J. Cardiol., 59*:725 (1987).

8. C. Falcone, S. DeServi, E. Poma, C. Campana, A. Scire, C. Montemartini, and G. Specchia. Clinical significance of exercise-induced silent myocardial ischemia in patients with coronary artery disease. *J. Am. Coll. Cardiol., 9*: 295 (1987).

9. S. O. Gottlieb, S. H. Gottlieb, S. C. Achuff, R. Baumgardner, E. D. Mellits, M. L. Weisfeldt, and G. Gerstenblith. Silent ischemia on Holter monitoring predicts mortality in high-risk postinfection patients. *JAMA 259*:1030 (1988).

10. P. F. Cohn. Silent myocardial ischemia in patients with a defective anginal warning system. *Am. J. Cardiol., 45*:697 (1980).

11. A. C. Cecchi, E. V. Dovellini, F. Marchi, P. Pucci, G. M. Santoro, and P. F. Fazzini. Silent myocardial ischemia during ambulatory electrocardiographic monitoring in patients with effort angina. *J. Am. Coll. Cardiol., 1*: 934 (1983).

12. D. Mulcahy, J. Keegan, P. Crean, et al. Silent myocardial ischemia in chronic stable angina: A study of its frequency and characteristics in 150 patients. *Br. Heart J., 60*:417 (1988).

13. S. O. Gottlieb, M. L. Weisfeldt, P. Ouyang, E. D. Mellits, and G. Gerstenblith. Silent ischemia predicts infarction and death during 2 year follow-up of unstable angina. *J. Am. Coll. Cardiol., 19*:756 (1987).

14. K. Nademanee, V. Intarachot, M. A. Josephson, D. Rieders, F. V. Mody, and B. N. Singh. Prognostic significance of silent myocardial ischemia in patients with unstable angina. *J. Am. Coll. Cardiol., 10*:1 (1987).

15. P. F. Cohn. Silent myocardial ischemia. *Ann. Intern. Med., 109*:312 (1988).

16. P. F. Cohn, G. W. Vetrovec, R. Nesto, and the Total Ischemia Awareness Program Investigators. The Nifedipine-Total Ischemia Awareness Program: A survey of painful and painless myocardial ischemia including results of anti-ischemic therapy. *Am. J. Cardiol.* (in press, March 1989).

17. B. Lown. Sudden cardiac death: The major challenge confronting contemporary cardiology. *Am. J. Cardiol., 43*:313 (1979).

18. L. H. Kuller. Sudden death: Definition and epidemiologic considerations. *Prog. Cardiovasc. Dis., 23*:1 (1980).

19. W. B. Kannel, L. A. Cupples, and R. B. D'Agostino. Sudden death risk in overt coronary heart disease: The Framingham Study. *Am. Heart J., 113*: 799 (1987).

20. S. Goldstein, S. V. Medendorp, J. R. Landis, R. A. Wolfe, R. Leighton, G. Ritter, C. M. Vasu, and A. Acheson. Analysis of cardiac symptoms preceding cardiac arrest. *Am. J. Cardiol., 58*:1195 (1986).

21. D. D. Savage, W. P. Castelli, S. J. Anderson, and W. B. Kannel. Sudden unexpected death during ambulatory electrocardiographic monitoring: The Framingham study. *Am. J. Med., 74*:148 (1983).

22. R. W. Harper, G. Kennedy, R. W. DeSanctis, and A. M. Hutter. The incidence and pattern of angina prior to acute myocardial infarction: A study of 577 cases. *Am. Heart J., 97*:178 (1979).

23. J. Midwall, J. Ambrose, A. Pichard, Z. Abedin, and M. V. Herman. Angina pectoris before and after infarction: Angiographic correlations. *Chest, 81*:6 (1982).

24. L. A. Pierard, C. Dubois, J-P. Smeets, J. Boland, J. Carlier, and H. E. Kulbertus. Prognostic significance of angina pectoris before first acutye myocardial infarction. *Am. J. Cardiol., 61*:984 (1988).

25. Y. Matsuda, H. Ogawa, K. Moritani, M. Matsuda, H. Naito, M. Matsuzaki, Y. Ikee, and R. Kusukawa. Effects of the presence or absence of preceding angina pectoris on left ventricular function after acute myocardial infarction. *Am. Heart J., 108*:955 (1984).

26. M. Matsuda, Y. Matsuda, H. Ogawa, K. Moritani, and R. Kusukawa. Angina pectoris before and during acute myocardial infarction: Relation to degree of physical activity. *Am. J. Cardiol., 55*:1255 (1985).

27. S. A. Samuel and P. F. Cohn. Myocardial infarction without a prior history of angina pectoris: A unique subset of coronary artery disease? (abstr). *Clin. Res., 33*:224A (1985).

6
Prevalence and Distinguishing Features of Silent Myocardial Infarctions

If one accepts the premise that myocardial ischemia can occur without symptoms, then it should not be surprising to learn that myocardial infarction can do the same. In fact, the literature on the latter predates the former, extending back over 75 years! Herrick was aware of it in his landmark paper published in 1912 [1] and anecdotal reports throughout the 1930s and 1940s maintained interest in this seeming paradox [2-5]. In 1954, Roseman reviewed the literature and analyzed 220 cases of this syndrome [6]. He concluded that its prevalence ranged from 20 to 60% of all infarc-

tions depending on the particular population surveyed either with electrocardiograms or by autopsy.

I. ELECTROCARDIOGRAPHIC STUDIES

One of the problems in assessing the frequency of silent infarctions is in
their definition. Unlike transient episodes of silent myocardial ischemia
that can be documented during exercise tests, radionuclide procedures,
Holter monitoring, etc., unrecognized infarctions are not witnessed at
the time they occur—except for the few that are detected via use of 24-hr
ambulatory electrocardiographic monitoring. Reliance on patients' mem-
ory of possible cardiac symptoms is not the best type of data, nor are physicians' office notes sufficient. In the final analysis, we are usually left with
electrocardiographic evidence of a myocardial infarction that occurred at
some point between two standard ECG examinations. Nevertheless, several groups have attempted to assess the frequency of this phenomenon
using ECG tracings. Probably the best example of these surveys is the
Framingham Study, a long-term prospective study of cardiovascular disease which began in 1948 in Framingham, Massachusetts, under the auspices of the National Institutes of Health. In this study, a standard cardiovascular examination was performed twice a year on 5209 subjects who
ranged from 30 to 62 years at time of entry into the study. Cardiovascular
end-points were noted on these examinations, as well as by reviewing admission lists at the town's hospital.

The initial report on unrecognized infarctions was published in 1970
[7] and supplemented in 1973 [8], 1984 [9], and 1986 [10]. The last report
represents a 26-year follow-up. At this time, over 28% of infarctions in
men and 35% in women were unrecognized (Figure 1). Of these, half were
truly silent, while in the other half some atypical symptoms were present
but were not sufficient for either the patient or physician to consider that
an infarction was occurring or had occurred. What this report also shows
is that these unrecognized infarctions were uncommon in patients with
prior angina. In a preliminary report concerning unrecognized infarction
in the age group 65-94 in the Framingham Study, Vokonas et al. [11] found
that 33% of infarctions in men and 36% in women were unrecognized.

Other groups have also studied silent infarctions. The Multiple Risk
Factor Intervention Trial (MRFIT) found 25% of infarctions to be unrecognized [12]. Another large study, that of the Western Collaborative
Group, found a 30% rate of unrecognized infarction [13]. Studies are not
confined to the United States. Medalie and Goldbourt [14] performed a

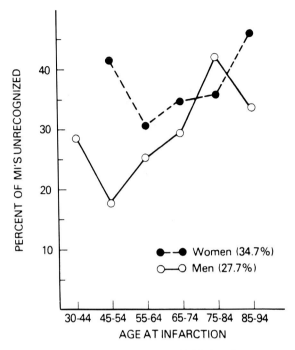

Figure 1 Proportion of myocardial infarctions unrecognized by age and sex in a 30-year follow-up in the Framingham Study. (From W. B. Kannel. *Cardiol. Clin.,* 4:583, 1986.)

prospective analysis in 9509 healthy government employees in Israel. Almost 40% of the subsequent 427 infarctions in this group were unrecognized. One difference between this study and that of the Framingham group was that these ECGs were read independently of prior tracings. This might tend to overestimate the number of unrecognized infarctions. Like the Framingham study, half of the unrecognized infarctions were totally silent. Also, like the Framingham study [15], increasing age and blood pressure were significantly associated with the development of unrecognized infarctions (Figure 2). In analyzing the age issue more closely, Aranow initially reported 68% of infarcts in an elderly population (64-100 years) were unrecognized [16]. He subsequently revised this figure to 21% in a prospective study (Table 1) when physicians were instructed to look more carefully for nonpain presentations (dyspnea, neurological symptoms, etc.) [17]. This is important, since symptoms due to the com-

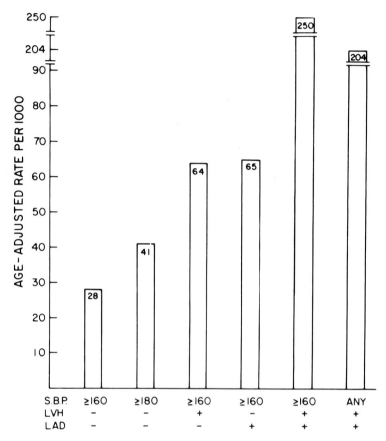

Figure 2   Five-year incidence of unrecognized (silent) myocardial infarction related to systolic blood pressure (SBP), left ventricular hypertrophy (LVH) and left axis deviation (LAD). (From J. H. Medalie and U. Goldbourt. *Ann. Intern. Med., 84*:256, 1976.)

plications of silent infarctions—such as pulmonary edema or dyspnea [18,19]—can be the first clue to the underlying problem.

II. AUTOPSY STUDIES

In addition to the reports cited earlier [2-5], more pertinent pathological studies have recently been made available comparing the extent of coronary narrowing and size of the healed infarct in these patients. Cabin and

Table 1 Prevalence of Presenting Symptoms of Recognized Acute Myocardial Infarction and of Unrecognized Healed Myocardial Infarction in 110 Documented Myocardial Infarctions in Elderly Patients

	n	(%)
Chest pain	24	(22)
Dyspnea	38	(35)
Neurological symptoms	20	(18)
Gastrointestinal symptoms	5	(4)
Unrecognized Q-wave myocardial infarction	23	(21)

Source: W. S. Aronow. Am. J. Cardiol., 60:1182, 1987.

Table 2 Clinical Findings in 33 Patients with Clinically Recognized and in 28 with Clinically Unrecognized Acute Myocardial Infarction (MI) and Healed Transmural Infarction at Necropsy

	Clinically recognized acute MI (33 patients)		Clinically unrecognized acute MI (28 patients)		
	n	%	n	%	p value
Age (yr)					
Mean	61	—	60	—	NS
Range	27-81	—	25-82	—	
Male-female ratio	25:8	—	21:7	—	NS
Angina pectoris	14	42	6	21	NS
Chronic congestive heart failure	14	42	9	32	NS
Systemic hypertension	11	33	12	43	NS
Diabetes mellitus (adult onset)	5	15	12	43	0.05
Mode of death					
Sudden	13	39	6	21	NS
Acute MI	8	24	7	25	NS
Chronic congestive heart failure	5	15	1	4	NS
Cardiac operation	2[a]	6	2[b]	7	NS
Cardiac catheterization	2	6	1	4	NS
Noncardiac	3	9	11	39	0.01

[a]Coronary artery bypass grafting in one and left ventricular aneurysmectomy in one.
[b]Coronary artery bypass grafting in both.
Source: H. S. Cabin and W. C. Roberts. Am. J. Cardiol., 50:677, 1982.

Roberts [20] studied 61 patients with a healed transmural myocardial infarction. Medical records were reviewed in details and the patients were divided into two groups according to the presence (33 patients) or absence (28 patients) of a clinical history of acute myocardial infarction. Patients with equivocal or inadequate histories were excluded. The group with unrecognized infarcts had a significantly higher prevalence of death from non-cardiac causes, posterior wall infarcts and small infarctions, as well as diabetes (Tables 2 and 3). However, the extent of narrowing of the coronary arteries was similar, as was the involvement of the various vessels (Table 4). The authors also addressed the question of whether patients

Table 3 Myocardial Infarct (MI) Size and Location in 33 Patients with and in 28 without a Clinical History of Acute MI and a Healed Transmural MI at Necropsy

Clinical history of acute MI	Patients (n)	MI size (%)		Number of patients with major (minor)[a] involvement of each left ventricular wall by MI			
		Range	Mean	Anterior	Posterior	Septal	Lateral
+	33	1-55	17	16 (1)	15 (3)	1 (12)	1 (14)
0	28	1-23	7	5 (1)	22 (1)	1 (8)	0 (9)
p value	—		0.001	0.01	0.025	NS	NS

[a]For each patient, major involvement refers to the left ventricular wall with the most scarring and minor involvement refers to 1 or more additional walls with scarring. In all but 3 patients the anterior or posterior wall of left ventricle was the site of major involvement.
Source: H. S. Cabin and W. C. Roberts. Am. J. Cardiol., 50:677, 1982.

Table 4 Number of Major Epicardial Coronary Arteries (CA) Narrowed 76-100% in Cross-Sectional Area (XSA) by Atherosclerotic Plaque in 33 Patients with and 28 Without a History of Acute Myocardial Infarction (MI) and a Healed Transmural MI at Necropsy

Clinical history acute MI	Patients (n)	Total CA (n)	Patients with CA narrowed 76-100% in XSA										Mean CA per patient narrowed 76-100%
			LM		LAD		LC		R		Totals		
+	33	132	6	18	32	97	23	70	32	97	93	70	2.8
0	28	112	8	29	24	86	21	75	28	100	81	72	2.9
p value	—	—	NS		NS		NS		NS		NS		NS

LAD = left anterior descending; LC = left circumflex; LM = left main; R = right.
Source: H. S. Cabin and W. C. Roberts. Am. J. Cardiol., 50:677, 1982.

with unrecognized infarcts had angina less frequently than did patients with symptomatic infarctions. Their results suggested this was the case, but the differences were not statistically significant.

III. MECHANISMS TO EXPLAIN THE ABSENCE OF PAIN: IS DIABETES MELLITUS A FACTOR?

In Chapter 1, we discussed cardiac pain pathways, and in Chapter 2, possible alterations in pain sensibility during silent myocardial ischemia. In addition, some investigators have studied pain mechanisms in patients

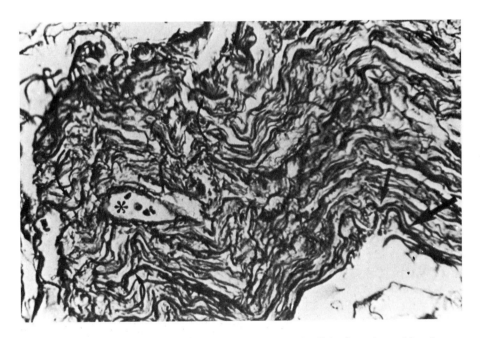

Figure 3 Abnormal appearance of a nerve fiber of a diabetic patient with painless myocardial infarction. Many fibers with hyperargentophilia, alterations of thickness and fragmentation (arrows). Abnormally small numbers of fibers. A vasa nervorum with normal wass (asterisk). Stain: trichrome and argentic impregnation. ×300. (From I. Faerman, E. Fraccio, J. Milei, R. Nunez, M. Jadzinsky, D. Fox, and M. Rapaport. *Diabetes, 26:*1147, 1977.)

with prior silent infarctions. Procacci et al. [21] studied 18 such subjects. They tested their cutaneous pain thresholds in the arm and found them to be significantly higher than in normals, but not higher than in patients with painful infarctions. They also studied upper-limb ischemia via cuff inflation and again found different onsets of pain and altered pain patterns compared to normals. They chose the arm because of the similar peripheral innervation found in "referred" cardiac pain.

These authors did not evaluate the effect of diabetes mellitus but others have. For example, Bradley and Schonfeld [22] reportd that 42 of 100 nondiabetic patients had painless infarctions compared with 6 of 100 nondiabetic patients. This relationship was confirmed in the previously cited

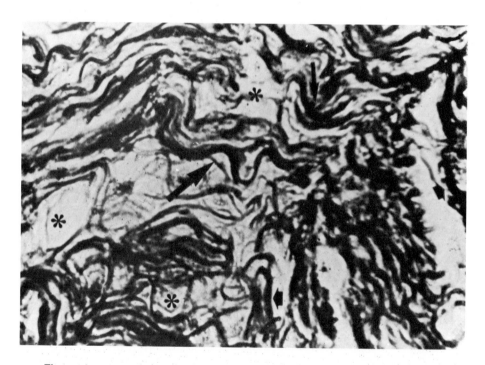

Figure 4 Abnormal nerve fiber in a diabetic patient with painless myocardial infarction. Note the spindle shape of many of the fibers (arrows), the interruption of fibers and the enlarged interfibrillar spaces (asterisks). Trichrome and argentic impregnation. × 1000. (From I. Faerman, E. Faccio, J. Milei, R. Nunez, M. Jadzinsky, D. Fox, and M. Rapaport. *Diabetes, 26*:1147, 1977.)

autopsy study of Cabin and Roberts [20]. As seen in Table 2, there was a significantly increased prevalence of diabetes mellitus among the patients in the unrecognized infarct group (43%) compared with those in the recognized infarct group. However, in two epidemiologic studies cited earlier [9,13], the association of diabetes with unrecognized myocardial infarction did not reach a statistically significant level.

Pathological involvement of the autonomic nervous system by diabetes was demonstrated by Faerman et al. [23]. Abnormal morphology was found in cardiac sympathetic and parasympathetic nerves (Figures 3-5). None of the changes were found in specimens taken from a control group. These findings of a visceral neuropathy may help to explain the absence of pain during transient ischemia, as well as during infarction. Raper et al.

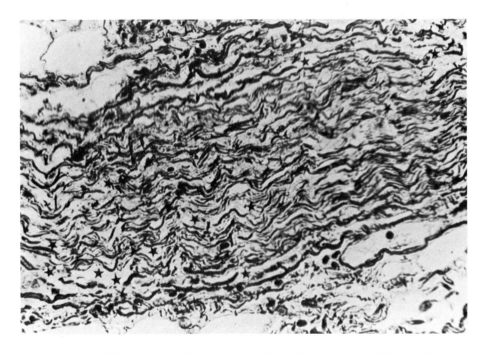

Figure 5 Diffuse abnormalities in a nerve fiber of the heart in a diabetic patient with painless myocardial infarction. Note the many fragmentations of the fibers (stars), hyperargentophilia and smaller number of fibers. Trichrome and argentic impregnation. ×300. (From I. Faerman, E. Faccio, J. Milei, R. Nunez, M. Jadzinsky, D. Fox, and M. Rapaport. *Diabetes, 26*:1147, 1977.)

[19] postulated that diabetes was responsible for painless infarction in one of four cases that they reported as presenting to the hospital with acute life-threatening cardiac illness. These patients came to the hospital because of complications of cardiac ischemia (such as pulmonary edema) but were pain-free.

Diabetes as a possible distinguishing feature of silent myocardial ischemia is discussed further in the next section of this book.

IV. CONCLUSIONS

One-quarter to one-third of myocardial infarctions are clinically unrecognized. Increasing age and hypertension are associated features. At autopsy the extent of coronary artery disease is similar to that seen with symptomatic infarctions. The etiology of painless infarctions is unclear, but the presence of diabetes appears to be a factor in some studies.

REFERENCES

1. J. B. Herrick. Clinical features of sudden obstruction of the coronary arteries. *J.A.M.A., 59*:2015 (1912).

2. J. A. Kennedy. The incidence of myocardial infarction without pain in autopsied cases. *Am. Heart J., 14*:703 (1937).

3. L. D. Boyde and S. C. Weblow. Coronary thrombosis without pain. *Am. J. Med. Sci., 194*:814 (1937).

4. L. E. Gorham and S. J. Martin. Coronary artery occlusion with and without pain. *Arch. Intern. Med., 112*:812 (1938).

5. W. D. Stroud and J. A. Wgner. Silent or atypical coronary occlusion. *Ann. Intern. Med., 15*:25 (1941).

6. M. D. Roseman. Painless myocardial infarction: A review of the literature and analysis of 220 cases. *Ann. Intern. Med., 41*:1 (1954).

7. W. B. Kannel, P. M. McNamara, M. Feinleib, et al. The unrecognized myocardial infarction: 14 year follow-up experience in the Framingham study. *Geriatrics, 25*:75 (1970).

8. J. R. Margolis, W. B. Kannel, M. Feinleib, et al. Clinical features of unrecognized myocardial infarction: 18 year follow-up: The Framingham study. *Am. J. Cardiol., 32*:1 (1973).

9. W. B. Kannel and R. D. Abbott. Incidence and prognosis of unrecognized myocardial infarction. Based on 26 years follow-up on the Framingham study. In *Silent Myocardial Ischemia* (W. Rutishauser and H. Roskamm, eds.), Springer-Verlag, Berlin, 1984, pp. 131-137.

10. W. B. Kannel. Silent myocardial ischemia and infarction: Insights from the Framingham Study. *Cardiol. Clin., 4*:583 (1986).

11. P. S. Vokonas, W. B. Kannel, and L. A. Cupples. Incidence and prognosis of unrecognized myocardial infarction in the elderly, The Framingham Study (abstr) *J. Am. Coll. Cardiol., 11*:51A, 1988.

12. R. H. Grimm, Jr., S. Tillinghast, K. Daniels, J. D. Neaton, S. Mascoli, R. Crow, M. Pritzker, and R. J. Prineas. Unrecognized myocardial infarction: Experience in the Multiple Risk Factor Intervention Trial (MRFIT). *Circulation, 75*(Suppl. II):6, 1987.

13. R. H. Rosenman, M. Friedman, C. D. Jenkins, et al. Clinically unrecognized infarction in the Western Collaborative Study. *Am. J. Cardiol., 19*:776 (1967).

14. J. H. Medalie and U. Goldbourt. Unrecognized myocardial infarction: Five-year incidence, mortality, and risk factors. *Ann. Intern. Med., 84*:526 (1976).

15. W. B. Kannel, A. L. Dannenberg, and R. D. Abbott. Unrecognized myocardial infarction and hypertension. The Framingham Study. *Am. Heart J., 109*: 581 (1985).

16. W. S. Aronow, L. Starling, F. Etienne, P. D'Alba, M. Edwards, N. H. Lee, and R. F. Parungao. Unrecognized Q-wave myocardial infarction in patients older than 64 years in a long-term health-care facility. *Am. J. Cardiol., 56*: 483 (1985).

17. W. S. Aronow. Prevalence of presenting symptoms of recognized acute myocardial infarction and of unrecognized healed myocardial infarction in elderly patients. *Am. J. Cardiol., 60*:1182 (1987).

18. J. E. Brush, H. S. Cabin, D. Wohlgelernter, G. L. Hammond, and L. S. Cohen. Ventricular septal rupture following a clinically unrecognized myocardial infarction. *Am. Heart J., 110*:667 (1985).

19. A. J. Raper, A. Hastillo, and W. J. Paulsen. The syndrome of sudden severe painless myocardial ischemia. *Am. Heart J., 107*:813 (1984).

20. H. S. Cabin and W. C. Roberts. Quantitative comparison of extent of coronary narrowing and size of healed myocardial infarct in 33 necropsy patients with clinically recognized and in 28 with clinically unrecognized ("silent") previous acute myocardial infarction. *Am. J. Cardiol., 50*:677 (1982).

21. P. Procacci, M. Zoppi, L. Padeletti, and M. Maresca. Myocardial infarction without pain. A study of the sensory function of the upper limbs. *Pain, 2*: 309 (1976).

22. R. F. Bradley and A. Schonfeld. Diminished pain in diabetic patients with myocardial infarction. *Geriatrics, 17*:322 (1962).

23. I. Faerman, E. Faccio, J. Milei, R. Nunez, M. Jadzinsky, D. Fox, and M. Rapaport. Autonomic neuropathy and painless myocardial infarction in diabetic patients: Histologic evidence of their relationship. *Diabetes, 26*:1147 (1977).

III
DETECTION OF ASYMPTOMATIC CORONARY ARTERY DISEASE

7

What Can Be Learned from Standard Diagnostic Procedures?

Considerable controversy surrounds the use of screening procedures for detecting coronary artery disease in asymptomatic populations [1-4]. The controversy concerns not only which procedures are most reliable, but also whether screening is even appropriate in the general population. We begin our review with a consideration of the more "routine" tests.

Standard diagnostic procedures for evaluating suspected coronary artery disease in persons *with* chest pain include history taking, physical examination, blood lipid and glucose determinations, the resting ECG, and chest X rays and related procedures. Exercise testing—with or without associated radioisotopic procedures—is usually the next step after these standard procedures and is discussed in subsequent chapters. Obviously, screening asymptomatic populations for the presence of coronary artery disease is a more difficult undertaking and in this regard not all of the above-mentioned procedures have the same value as they do in patients with chest pain syndromes.

I. HISTORY TAKING

This is of limited value since, by definition, the individual to be screened has no symptoms. (This, of course, does not include patients now asymptomatic who have experienced a prior infarction.) At times, cardiologists will clearly recognize anginal equivalents that have been misdiagnosed by the patients (or their physicians) as gastrointestinal or neuromuscular complaints. Some complaints may or may not reflect underlying heart disease. "Breathlessness" is one such symptom that must be carefully considered as having a cardiac basis, since true dyspnea can be a sign of left ventricular failure due to ischemia [5]. Perhaps the most important information that truly asymptomatic individuals can provide, however, relates to their family history and/or their own known coronary risk factors.

If a member of the individual's immediately family (i.e., parents, grandparents, aunts, uncles) died of cardiac (or unknown) causes or developed a myocardial infarction or angina before the age of 55, this should alert the cardiologist or internist to the possibility of laent coronary atherosclerosis. Since much of a "positive family history" is due to the prevalence of the three most important genetically detemined risk factors (hypertension, diabetes mellitus, hypercholesterolemia), patients should then be queried directly about the presence of these factors in their relatives—and themselves. Although cigarette smoking is not an inherited problem, smoking is another risk factor that can be part of a positive family history since patients who smoke encourage their children to do likewise merely by setting an example.

II. PHYSICAL EXAMINATION

Unless the patient has experienced a prior myocardial infarction with resulting left ventricular asynergy and its characteristic cardiac findings, the physical examination is usually negative. A fourth heart sound may be present even in individuals without prior infarctions, but this is too nonspecific a finding to be used by itself to diagnose coronary artery disease. The reliability of the "ear lobe crease" sign is also uncertain.

III. BLOOD TESTS

Abnormal blood glucose or lipid levels are recognized risk factors for the development of coronary artery disease. Whether they can be used as *indicators* of asymptomatic coronary artery disease is less clear.

Epidemiologic studies—such as that in Framingham, Massachusetts— have clearly shown the increased risk associated with increasing levels of serum cholesterol [6]. Other studies have examined the ratio of total cholesterol to high density lipoprotein (HDL) cholesterol. Williams et al. [7] studied 2568 asymptomatic men and found that a ratio of 4.0 or less identified a group with a very low prevalence of disease, whereas a ratio of 8.0 or above identified a very high-risk group in relation to future cardiac events. Serum lipid levels have also been used to aid in the selection of subjects for coronary arteriography. Uhl et al. [8] found a ratio greater than 6.0 generated an odds ratio of 172/1 based on coronary angiographic results in 132 asymptomatic airmen with a positive exercise test. Only 2 of the 16 with coronary artery disease had a ratio less than 6.0, whereas only 4/102 persons with normal coronary angiographic findings had a ratio greater than 6.0. The ratio was a better discriminator than total cholesterol or HDL cholesterol levels (Figures 1 and 2). The value of this ratio was recently confirmed in a preliminary report by Houck [9] in screening over 11,000 Air Force personnel. In another preliminary report, Kwiterovich et al. [10] investigated the elevated apoprotein levels of coronary artery disease in an asymptomatic population. Apoproteins are associated with cholesterol transport, and the major apoprotein B of low-density lipoproteins has previously been shown to be elevated in symptomatic individuals. In their report, Kwiterovich et al. studied plasma levels of various types of cholesterol and apoproteins in 68 asymptomatic siblings of 40 patients with premature coronary artery disease. Of the 19 siblings with a positive stress-thallium test, 10 had elevated apoprotein B levels. Bivariate analysis showed that apoprotein B was significantly more sensitive in this regard than other cholesterol and apoprotein measurements. As this study suggests, the presence of single or multiple risk factors combined with abnormal exercise responses can also improve predictive value for coronary artery disease. This is discussed at greater length in Chapters 9 and 10.

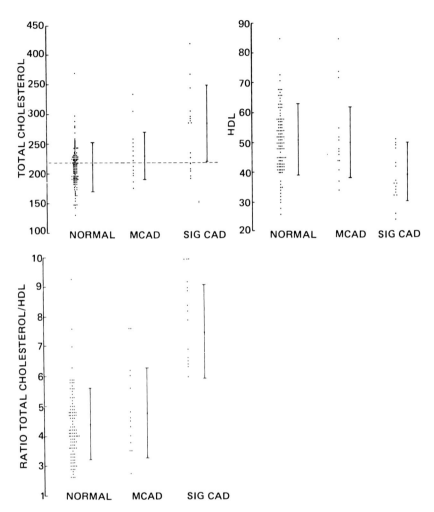

Figure 1   Values for total cholesterol, HDL cholesterol, and cholesterol/HDL cholesterol ratio in each of the patients plotted according to angiographic classification (normal, minimal coronary artery disease [MCAD] and significant coronary artery disease [SIG CAD]). An arbitrary cutoff value for total cholesterol of 220 mg/100 ml is represented by the dotted line. Total cholesterol and HDL cholesterol levels did not discriminate between those with significant coronary artery disease and those with normal coronary angiograms. A cholesterol/HDL cholesterol ratio greater than 6.0 was the best discriminator. (From G. S. Uhl, R. G. Troxler, J. R. Hickman, Jr., and D. Clark. *Am. J. Cardiol., 48*:903, 1981.)

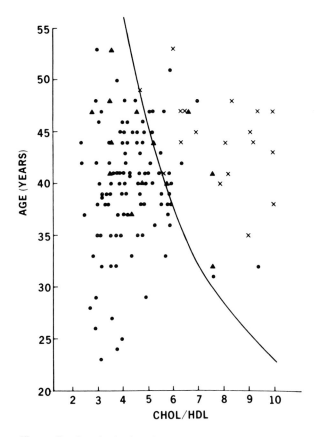

Figure 2 Graph plotting the cholesterol (CHOL)/HDL cholesterol ratio versus age for each patient who underwent cardiac catheterization. The ratio and age appear to be independent risk factors. The solid line plots the equation: age × (total cholesterol/HDL cholesterol) = 230. It demonstrates that a simple equation can separate normal subjects from patients with significant coronary artery disease (CAD). ● = normal; ▲ = minimal CAD; x = significant CAD. (From G. S. Uhl, R. G. Troxler, J. R. Hickman, Jr., and D. Clark. *Am. J. Cardiol., 48*:903, 1981.)

IV. THE RESTING ELECTROCARDIOGRAM

The standard baseline ECG obtained at rest is of value if it shows unequivocal evidence of new or old myocardial infarction. In totally asymptomatic individuals, one assumes the infarct was either silent, or painless enough not to warrant concern by the patient and/or his physician at the

Table 1   Angiographic Findings in 111 Aircrewmen with an Abnormal Exercise Electrocardiogram Grouped According to Annual Rest Electrocardiographic (ECG) Findings

Annual rest ECG	n	Mean age (%)	Significant angiographic coronary disease (%)
Normal	34	44	23.5
Previous ST-T change but current ECG normal	21	43	23.8
Low amplitude T waves	24	42	25.0
St segment abnormal	32	44	46.9

Source: V. Froelicher, A. J. Thompson, R. Wolthius, et al. *Am. J. Cardiol., 23*:32, 1977.

time. The finding of ST abnormalities alone suggests that underlying coronary artery disease will be found in a relatively small number of subjects, but when combined with a positive exercise test, the predictive value increases to nearly 50%, which is higher than that observed with T wave changes alone (Table 1) [11]. Joy and Trump [12] concluded from their study of 103 asymptomatic men with minor ST segment abnormalities that the predictive value for coronary artery disease for these changes alone was about 8%, whereas it was 44% when combined with a positive exercise test. Changes with hyperventilation were not as impressive and these could not be used to separate presumably normal persons from those with coronary artery disease. This was also true of the U.S. Air Force studies [11]. In other Air Force patients, the prevalence rate of coronary artery disease was 22% in asymptomatic airmen with new left bundle branch block and 18% in right bundle branch block [11].

Ventricular premature beats—either on resting ECGs or on Holter monitors—are not in themselves regarded as indicators, or predictors, of coronary artery disease if other evidence of organic heart disease is lacking [13].

Another approach to the ECG is computer analysis of the first and second integral of the voltage versus time (the "cardiointegram"). In a preliminary report [14] predictive accuracy was 74% in 186 patients who had also undergone cardiac catheterization and had normal resting ECGs. This device may be useful as a screening tool if results are confirmed in the future.

V. CHEST X RAYS AND RELATED PROCEDURES

The chest X ray is usually normal in this type of patient unless a prior infarction has occurred, or an ischemic cardiomyopathy has developed. Fluoroscopic screening for coronary artery disease (via detection of coronary artery calcification) is simple, rapid and inexpensive, but its reliability has been questioned, especially in older patients. In a preliminary study [15], Rifkin et al. studied 184 asymptomatic subjects with fluoroscopy and coronary angiography. They found that coronary artery calcification was a strong marker for coronary artery stenosis in subjects under the age of 50 years but is a weak marker for those over the age of 60 years. Some groups have used the combination of fluoroscopy and exercise testing as screening markers in asymptomatic populations. We will consider this in Chapter 10. Echocardiograms and radionuclide ventriculography are also considered in Chapter 10 as adjuncts to the exercise test, since stress-related abnormalities of left ventricular wall motion are much more common than resting abnormalities in asymptomatic persons. One instrument that has been reported in a preliminary study to detect abnormal left ventricular function at rest is the cardiokymograph. The cardiokymograph is an electronic device that produces a representation of regional left ventricular wall motion. Zoltnick et al. [16] studied 287 asymptomatic subjects. They found an abnormal cardiokymograph to have a predictive value of 50%, equaling that of stress testing.

VI. CONCLUSIONS

Standard clinical procedures are of limited value as indicators of asymptomatic coronary artery disease, though coronary risk factors can help predict who will *subsequently* develop coronary artery disease.

REFERENCES

1. G. S. Uhl and V. Froelicher. Screening for asymptomatic coronary artery disease. *J. Am. Coll. Cardiol., 1*:946 (1983).

2. R. Detrano and V. Froelicher. A logical approach to screening for coronary artery disease. *Ann. Intern. Med., 106*:846 (1987).

3. D. S. Berman, A. Rozanski, and S. B. Knoebel. The detection of silent ischemia: cautions and precautions. *Circulation, 75*:101 (1987).

4. R. H. Helfant, L. W. Klein, and J. B. Agarwal. Role of cardiac testing in an era of proliferating technology and cost containment. *J. Am. Coll. Cardiol., 9*:1194 (1987).

5. P. G. F. Nixon and L. J. Freeman. What is the meaning of angina pectoris today? *Am. Heart J., 114*:1542 (1987).

6. W. B. Kannell, W. P. Castelli, and T. Gordon. Cholesterol in the prediction of atherosclerotic disease: New perspective based on the Framingham Study. *Ann. Intern. Med., 90*:85 (1979).

7. P. Williams, D. Robinson, and A. Bailey. High density lipoprotein and coronary risk factors in normal men. *Lancet, 1*:72 (1979).

8. G. S. Uhl, R. G. Troxler, J. R. Hickman, Jr., and D. Clark. Angiographic correlation of coronary artery disease with high density lipoprotein cholesterol in asymptomatic men. *Am. J. Cardiol., 48*:903 (1981).

9. P. D. Houck. Epidemiology of total-cholesterol-to-HDL (ratio) in 11,669 Air Force personnel and coronary artery anatomy in 305 health aviators. *J. Am. Coll. Cardiol., 11*:222A (1988).

10. P. O. Kwiterovich, D. M. Becker, T. Pearson, D. J. Fintel, P. Bachorik, and A. Sniderman. HyperapoB is a potent predictor of occult coronary artery disease in asymptomatic relatives (abstr). *Circulation, 70*(Suppl 11):313 (1984).

11. V. Froelicher, A. J. Thompson, R. Wolthuis, et al. Angiographic findings in asymptomatic aircrewmen with electrocardiographic abnormalities. *Am. J. Cardiol., 39*:32 (1977).

12. M. Joy and D. W. Trump. Significance of minor ST segment and T wave changes in the resting electrocardiogram of asymptomatic subjects. *Br. Heart J., 45*:48 (1981).

13. A. J. Moss. Clinical significance of ventricular arrhythmias in patients with and without coronary artery disease. *Prog. Cardiovasc. Dis., 23*:33 (1980).

14. L. E. Teichholz, M. Y. Steinmetz, D. Escher, M. V. Herman, D. V. Mahony, M. H. Ellestad, and S. Naimi. The cardiointegram: Detection of coronary artery disease in patients with normal resting electrocardiograms (abstr). *J. Am. Coll. Cardiol., 3*:598 (1984).

15. R. D. Rifkin, B. F. Uretsky, S. C. Sharma, E. D. Polland, D. A. Pietro, G. V. R. K. Sharma, P. S. Readdy, and A. F. Parisi. Fluroscopic screening for coronary artery disease (abstr). *Circulation, 70*(Suppl 11):281 (1984).

16. J. M. Zoltick, J. Patton, J. Vogel, W. Daniels, J. L. Bedynek, and J. E. Davia. Cardiovascular screening evaluation to test for coronary artery disease in asymptomatic males over the age of 40 (abstr.). *J. Am. Coll. Cardiol., 1*:638 (1982).

8

Ambulatory Electrocardiography (Holter Monitoring)

Along with the exercise test, the 24-48-hr ambulatory electrocardiogram (popularly known as the Holter monitor after its inventor) has become closely identified with the documentation of silent myocardial ischemia. No longer is this device used only for the detection of arrhythmias, but rather it has gained increasing attention as the best way of detecting transient myocardial ischemia during daily activities. The validity of this approach has been confirmed in a host of studies.

103

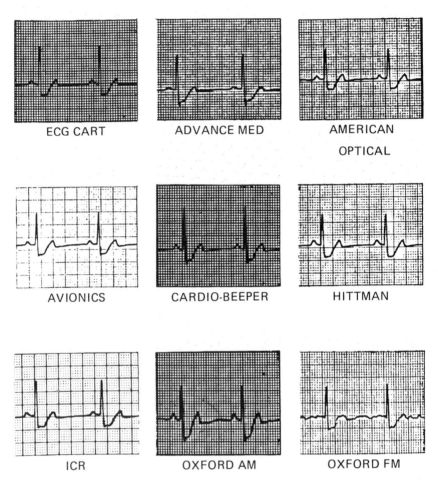

ECG CART   ADVANCE MED   AMERICAN
                                                     OPTICAL

AVIONICS   CARDIO-BEEPER   HITTMAN

ICR   OXFORD AM   OXFORD FM

Figure 1 The representative output from one record/transmitter and one scan-ner/receiver of the input of the modified ECG simulator with 4-mm flat-line ST segment depression of 80msec duration. Note the output from an HP 12-lead ECG cart (model 1541A) used as the standard. Note that the American Optical, Avionics and ICR systems gave good reproduction of the signal. Although the Hittman system reproduced the ST segment there was some attenuation of the terminal S wave. The Oxford AM gave considerably more than 4.0-mm ST seg-ment depression. Advance Med and Cardio-Beeper had slightly upsloping ST seg-ments. Note the baseline noise present on Oxford FM which limits clinical inter-pretation. (From D. A. Bragg-Remschel, C. M. Anderson, and R. A. Winkle. *Am. Heart J., 103*:20, 1982.)

I. TECHNICAL CONSIDERATIONS

The issue of whether or not ST segment changes recorded on Holter monitors are reliable indicators of myocardial ischemia is no longer as controversial as it once was, i.e., when continuous ambulatory monitoring was
introduced in the 1960s. There are still problem areas, however. What-
ever the ECG recording procedure employed—Holter, exercise tests, etc.—it
is well known that ST segments are labile and notoriously susceptible to
hyperventilation, electrolyte abnormalities, drugs, etc., but there have
also been specific criticisms concerning the ambulatory ECG. Some of
these involve technical considerations in recording of the electrocardiographic signal. The American Heart Association [1] has recommended a
flat amplitude signal for frequency responses between 0.1 and 80 Hz, but
many of the amplitude modulated (AM) ambulatory ECG monitoring

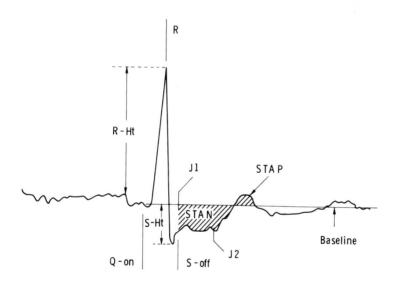

Figure 2 Diagram showing the variables identified and measured for each cardiac cycle by a computer system. J_1 = J joint; J_2 = level of the ST segment 60msec
after the J point; R = R wve; R-Ht = R wave amplitude; S-Ht = S wave amplitude; Q-on = onset on Q wave; S-off = end of S wave; STAN = ST segment
negative area; STAP = ST segment positive area. Heart rate is calculated from
the RR interval. (From A. Gallino, S. Chierchia, G. Smith, M. Croom, M. Morgan, C. Marchesi, and A. Maseri. *J. Am. Coll. Cardiol., 4*:245, 1984.)

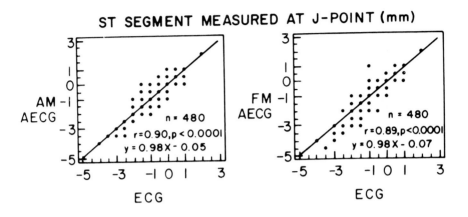

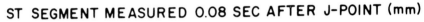

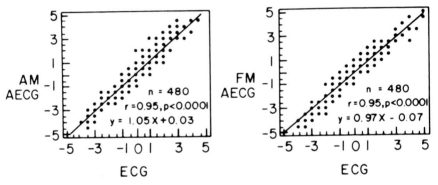

Figure 3   Reproduction of the ST segment measured at the J point and 0.08 second after the J point by amplitude-modulated (AM) and frequency-modulated (FM) systems, compared with the standard direct-writing electrocardiogram (1 mV = 10 mm). Note: Each point may represent more than 1 determination. AECG = ambulatory electrocardiogram. (From T. L. Shook, C. W. Balke, P. W. Kotilainen, M. Hubelbank, A. P. Selwyn, and P. H. Stone. *Am. J. Cardiol., 60*:895, 1987.)

systems amplify low-frequency information normally present in the ST segment. This can have the effect of overestimating the degree of ST segment depression relative to the height of the R wave. In addition to the concerns with frequency response curves, there is also the specific monitor to consider. Different systems will record standardized ST segment signals with different wave forms (Figure 1). Analysis of Holter types can also present difficulties. Recently developed computer programs for detecting transient ST changes appear to offer the best ways of analyzing the Holter tapes [2] (Figure 2).

Since most of the equipment in use at hospitals and diagnostic laboratories is of the AM type, it is important that physicians have assurances that the report they receive is accurate. Lambert et al. [3] have provided such assurances for the reliability of AM devices in their study of low-frequency requirements for recording ischemic ST segment abnormalities. Their conclusion—that current AM models are as reliable as the "gold standard" frequency modulated (FM) systems—has been confirmed by Shook et al. [4] in a different study protocol (Figures 3 and 4). Ironically, as this issue appears to be resolved, another has emerged. A new type of

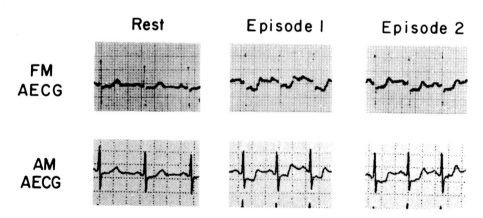

Figure 4 Representative simultaneous frequency-modulated (FM) and amplitude-modulated (AM) Holter recording during episodes of out-of-hospital ischemic ST-segment change. AECG = ambulatory electrocardiogram. (From T. L. Shook, C. W. Balke, P. W. Kotilainen, M. Hubelbank, A. P. Selwyn, and P. H. Stone. *Am. J. Cardiol., 60*:895, 1987.)

Holter monitor using real-time analysis has been developed. This has presented a new set of problems, as discussed by Kennedy and Wiens [5]. In the final analysis, the use of these real-time devices depends on validation studies comparing the devices with conventional AM and FM monitors, as has been done with one such system [6,7].

II. CORRELATION BETWEEN HOLTER STUDIES AND CORONARY ARTERIOGRAPHY

Stern and Tzivoni [8] were the first to demonstrate ST segment abnormalities on Holter monitoring in a series of 80 patients with chest pain syndromes, normal resting electrocardiograms and normal exercise tests. Thirty-seven of the eighty patients had ischemic ST segment abnormalities (either elevation or depression) on their ambulatory recordings. Many of these episodes were unaccompanied by pain (Figure 5). In the initial 12-month follow-up period, 1 of these 37 patients developed a myocardial infarction; 23 others developed increasing chest pain or further ECG changes suggestive of coronary artery disease. Coronary arteriography was not performed in any of these patients. In another study, Stern and Tzivoni [9] studied 140 patients with chronic ischemic heart disease documented by anginal histories or myocardial infarctions. Ninety-seven of the one hundred forty patients had ST segment abnormalities during their daily activities. Some individuals (24%) had more ischemic episodes during sleep, while others (38%) had less episodes. In yet another of their early studies [10], this group correlated the results of ambulatory monitoring with coronary arteriography: ambulatory ECGs identified nearly 80% of patients with angiographically documented coronary artery disease. The false-positive rate (abnormal Holter findings with normal coronary arteriograms) was only 13%.

In the late 1970s, other groups also attempted to correlate ambulatory ECGs with the results of coronary arteriograms. Crawford and colleagues [11] studied 70 patients (39 with and 31 without coronary artery disease) with 24-hr ambulatory monitors, exercise stress tests, as well as coronary arteriography. Twenty-four of the thirty-nine patients (62%) with coronary artery disease had ischemic ST segment abnormalities on the 24-hr monitors. This compared to 26 patients (or 67%) who had positive stress tests. By contrast, in the 31 patients free of coronary artery disease, 19 (61%) had no ischemic abnormalities on 24-hr monitoring. The exercise stress test was negative in 23 of the 31 subjects (75%).

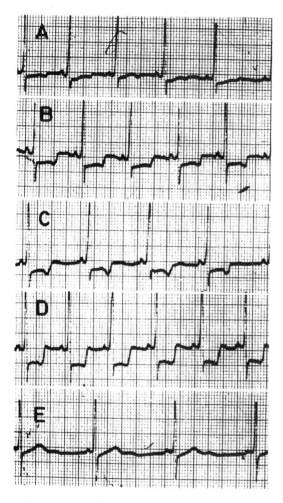

Figure 5 An example of the ST-T changes observed during 24-hr ambulatory ECG monitoring in a 56-year-old man. Slight ST-T abnormalities were noted during most of the day (panel A); increasing degrees of ST segment depression were observed after meals (panel B), at rest (panel C) and during walking (panel D). Only during sleep at night (panel E) was the ECG normal. Although the patient had apparent evidence of myocardial ischemia as shown in panels B, C, and D, the only experienced pain during walking (panel D). (From S. Stern and D. Tzivoni, *Am. Heart J.*, *91*:820, 1976.)

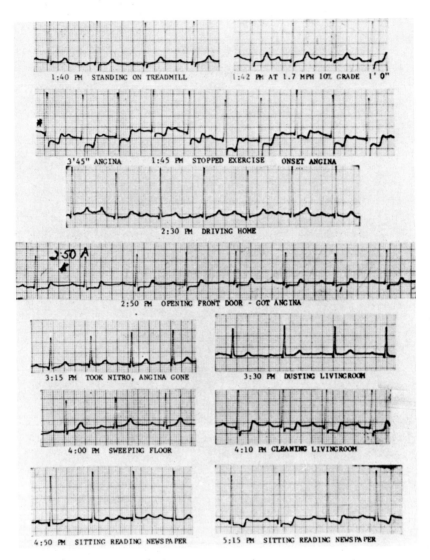

Figure 6   Another example of ST-T changes observed on ambulatory monitoring in a building manager. ECG changes occurred on an exercise test, during work, and at rest, but were not always accompanied by pain. (From S. J. Schang and C. J. Pepine. *Am. J. Cardiol., 39*:396, 1977.)

III. HOLTER MONITORING AND SILENT MYOCARDIAL ISCHEMIA

Most of the studies cited above dealt peripherally with the issue of silent myocardial ischemia. The first Holter study to specifically evaluate the significance of asymptomatic episodes was that of Schang and Pepine [12]. Twenty patients with angiographically confirmed coronary artery disease and positive exercise tests were each monitored for several 10-hr periods over the course of 16 months. In the total of 2826 hr of technically adequate recordings, 411 episodes of transient ST segment abnormalities were documented (Figure 6). Of the 411 episodes, 308 (or 75%) were asymptomatic. Most of these occurred during sleep, sitting or periods of slow walking and at heart rates very much less than those at which patients complained of angina during their stress tests. Schang and Pepine indirectly "proved" that the silent ST segment episodes were truly ischemic by markedly reducing their occurrence with the frequent, prophylactic use of nitrate preparations. This was an important feature of their study, since, as noted previously, considerable criticism had been directed toward the use of the ST segment as a marker of ischemia.

However, it was not until the study published by Deanfield and co-workers [13] appeared that this criticism abated. This study and its successor [14] succeeded in refuting much of the skepticism concerning the occurrence and significance of symptomatic versus asymptomatic episodes. In 30 patients with stable angina and positive exercise tests, ambulatory ST segment monitoring was used to record episodes of transient ischemia during daily life. All patients had four consecutive days of monitoring, and in 20 patients long-term variability was evaluated by repeated 48-hr monitoring and exercise testing over an 18-month period. Of the 1934 episodes of horizontal or downsloping ST segment depression, only 470 (or 24%) were accompanied by angina—a figure almost identical to that of Schang and Pepine in their study published 6 years earlier. Physiologic validation of the ST segment change was an especially important part of their second study [14], which included 34 patients. That ischemia could occur without angina was documented by positron tomography (see Figures 14 and 15 in Chapter 4) with the occurrence of ST segment depression being consistently underestimated by symptoms. Heart rate increase was not common (Figure 7), suggesting that transient increases in coronary vasomotor tone were a major contributor to myocardial ischemia—with or without symptoms—during daily activities.

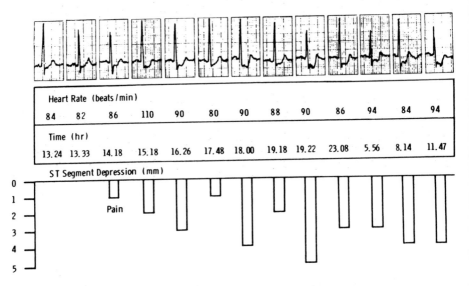

Figure 7 Typical 24-hr ambulatory electrocardiographic recording showing 11 episodes of ST depression, only one of which was accompanied by angina. The episodes occurred throughout day and night and lasted for up to 40 min. (From J. E. Deanfield, P. Ribiero, K. Oakley, S. Krikler, and A. P. Selwyn. *Am. J. Cardiol., 54*:1195, 1984.)

Table 1 Ischemic Episodes During Holter Monitoring (39 patients)

Patients (no.)	Total	Episodes (no.)	
		Symptomatic	Asymptomatic
7	—	0	—
8	25	25	—
15	105	29	76
9	40	—	40
Total	170	54	116

Source: A. C. Cecci, E. V. Dovellini, F. Marchi, P. Pucci, C. M. Santoro, and P. F. Fazzini. *J. Am. Coll. Cardiol., 1*:934, 1983.

Table 2 24 Hour Holter Monitoring: Duration of Ischemia Attacks and Magnitude of Maximal ST Depression

	Patients (no.)	Episodes (no.)	Type of episodes	Duration of episodes	Mean magnitude of maximal ST depression
All patients	32	54	Sympatomatic	7' ± 5'42"	3.3 ± 1.7 mm
		116	Asymptomatic	4'12" ± 2'30"	2.5 ± 1 mm
		Total 170		(p < 0.001)	(p < 0.001)
Patients who experienced					
only symptomatic	8	25	Symptomatic	5'12" ± 3'50"	2.3 ± 0.9 mm
or asymptomatic episodes	9	40	Asymptomatic	4'33" ± 3'	2.7 ± 1.2 mm
		Total 65		(p > 0.05)	(p > 0.05)
Patients who exhibited					
both symptomatic and	15	29	Symptomatic	8'36" ± 6'35"	4.3 ± 1.7 mm
asymptomatic episodes		76	Asymptomatic	4'06" ± 2'15"	2.4 ± 1.0 mm
		Total 105		(p < 0.001)	(p < 0.001)

Source: A. C. Cecci, E. V. Dovellini, F. Marchi, P. Pucci, C. M. Santoro, and P. F. Fazzini. *J. Am. Coll. Cardiol..* 1:934, 1983.

Other studies have confirmed the frequency of silent ischemic episodes in patients with classic exertion-induced angina pectoris, as well as their occurrence at lower heart rates. Cecci and colleagues [15] also found the number of silent episodes to outnumber the symptomatic ones. In their study of 39 patients with exertion-induced angina, they performed 24-hr Holter monitoring in addition to exercise testing. Coronary artery disease was confirmed by coronary arteriography in 31 patients, and 16 patients had a prior myocardial infarction. Of the 39 patients, 32 had ST depression during ambulatory monitoring (Table 1). Fifteen of the thirty-two patients had both symptomatic and asymptomatic episodes (with symptomatic episodes being three times as frequent); in this study the duration and degree of ST segment depression was greater during the asymptomatic episodes (Table 2). Deanfield et al. [13] noted that most of the asymptomatic episodes were short, while the symptomatic ones were just as likely to be long rather than short (Figure 8). The myocardial perfusion defects appeared similar, however. Cecci et al. [15] also reported that patients who took longer to register chest pain during treadmill stress

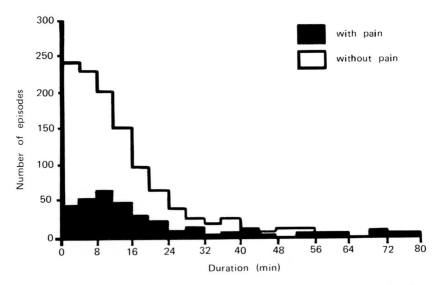

Figure 8 Histogram showing duration of symptomatic and asymptomatic episodes of ST depression. (From J. E. Deanfield, A. P. Selwyn, S. Chierchia, A. Maseri, P. Ribiero, S. Krikler, and M. Morgan. *Lancet, 2*:753, 1983.)

Table 3 Results of Stress Testing and Holter Monitoring

Stress Testing			Holter Monitoring		
			Episodes (no.)		
Patients (no.)	Finding	Patients (no.)	Symptomatic	Asymptomatic	Ratio between symptomatic and asymptomatic episodes
11	Angina precedes or coincides with ST depression	11	27	17	1:0.62
10	ST depression precedes angina by 10 to 60 seconds	8	11	12	1:1.09
18	ST depression precedes angina by more than 60 seconds	13	16	87	1:5.43

Source: A. C. Cecci, E. V. Dovellini, F. Marchi, P. Pucci, C. M. Santoro, and P. F. Fazzini. *J. Am. Coll. Cardiol., 1*:934, 1983.

testing had a greater ratio of symptomatic to painless episodes of myocardial ischemia on 24-hr monitoring (Table 3). Their studies suggested
that the severity of the ischemic episode, i.e., the amount of myocardium
at jeopardy, is an important factor in determining whether a specific ischemic episode would be symptomatic or not (see also Chapter 4). By
contrast, Kunkes et al. [16] reported that patients with multivessel disease (and presumably *more* myocardium at jeopardy) had a higher frequency of silent ischemic episodes than did patients with one-vessel disease (Figure 9).

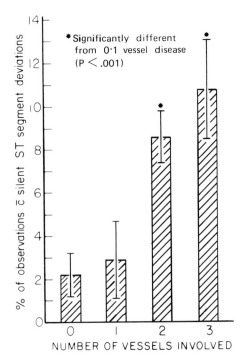

Figure 9   Correlation of silent ST segment deviations with the extent for coronary artery disease. Hatched bars represent the percentage of observation with
silent ST segment deviations on the ambulatory ECG for each grade of coronary
artery disease. Note how this percentage increases with the extent of coronary artery disease. * = significantly different from 0-1-vessel disease ($p < 0.001$). (From
S. H. Kunkes, A. D. Pichard, H. Smith, Jr., R. Gorlin, M. V. Herman, and J.
Kupersmith. Am. Heart H., 100:813, 1980.)

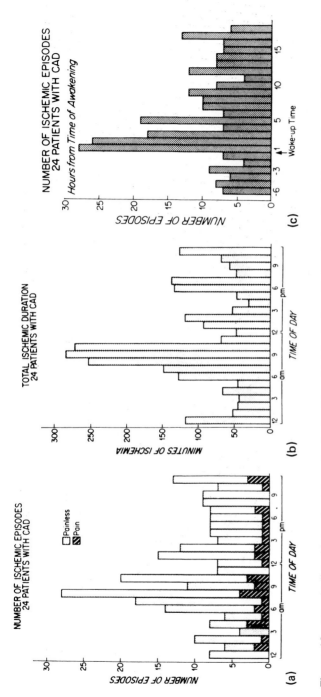

Figure 10 Hourly distribuiton of number of episodes (a) and total minutes of ischemic duration (b) in 24 patients with ischemic ST segment depression. There is a significant peak of ischemic activity between 6 A.M. and 12 noon. When the number of episodes is corrected for the time of waking (c), the peak density of ischemic activity occurs immediately upon rising. (From M. B. Rocco, J. Barry, S. Campbell, E. Nabel, E. F. Cook, L. Goldman, and A. P. Selwyn. *Circulation, 75:*392, 1987.)

117

Table 4 Results in All Patients and Day-to-Day Variations

Pt	Results of 3 monitoring days				% maximal day-to-day variations			
	No. of episodes	Total duration of ST↓ (min)	Maximal ST↓ (min)	HR at beginning of ST↓ (beats/min)	No. of episodes (%)	Duration of ST↓ (%)	Maximal ST↓ (%)	HR at beginning of ST↓ (%)
1	28	121	1.5	75	36	78	0	16.7
2	12	280	2	87	60	48	0	3.3
3	16	132	3.5	85	43	25	43	13.3
4	23	609	6	85	33	75	17	10.5
5	13	673	6	85	20	90	17	10.5
6	12	147	2	85	60	58	25	15
7	7	136	3	90	33	48	50	14.3
8	9	60	4	85	50	56	62	7.6
9	22	52	6	95	44	83	75	5
10	18	44	1.5	93	17	29	33	7
11	25	190	3	95	22	43	33	0
12	16	159	3	100	43	62	25	4.8
13	12	126	2	90	40	30	38	8.2
14	29	329	4	77	10	39	33	8.3
15	12	78	1.5	75	40	57	37	8.5
16	31	268	4	78	25	48	14	13.3
17	38	390	3.5	75	26	23	33	8.5
18	19	212	4.5	90	29	23	22	5.3
19	29	366	3.5	88	27	66	30	12
20	18	200	3.5	80	56	39	29	8.1
Mean	19.5	228.6	3.4	81.4	35.9	51.1	30.8	9

HR = heart rate; ↓ = depression.

Source: D. Tzivoni, A. Gavish, J. Benhorin, S. Banai, A. Keren, and S. Stern. *Am. J. Cardiol.*, *60*:1003, 1987.

As more and more studies using the Holter monitor have been published, it is apparent that episodes involving ST elevation often have similar characteristics to episodes involving ST depression in regard to heart rate, duration of ischemia, etc. [17], that there is a circadian variation in these episodes, with most coming after arousal in the morning [18] (Figure 10), perhaps related to enhanced platelet aggregation [19], that silent events are also common in patients with unstable angina [20] and that Holter monitoring is useful in assessing success of coronary angioplasty [21]. The day to day variability in these events must be considered [22,23], however (Table 4). This will be discussed further when therapy is discussed in subsequent chapters. At that time we will also consider the use of Holter monitoring in multicenter trials, for example, the Total Ischemia Awareness Program (TIAP) [24] that evaluated the significance of silent ischemia in clinical practice.

The use of ambulatory monitoring for detecting silent ischemia via ST segment abnormalities in asymptomatic persons without coronary arteriographic evidence of coronary artery disease has been questioned very strenuously. When Armstrong and Morris [25] evaluated 50 asymptomatic middle-aged men with treadmill exercise tests and ambulatory ECG monitoring and found evidence of "ischemic" ST segment changes in 15 of the 50 men (30%), they concluded that these were false-positive responses, similar to those observed in cases of mitral valve prolapse or neurocirculatory asthenia or in any condition where the autonomic nervous system can be overactive. Others [26,27] have also reported ST segment changes in presumably healthy men, but Deanfield et al. [28] found significant depression only rarely. When asymptomatic patients with coronary artery disease are studied, Holter monitoring commonly detects episodes of silent ischemia [29-31]. In some of the patients, the disease is quite extensive. Diabetics appear especially prone to silent ischemia [32], presumably as a reflection of their high incidence of coronary artery disease and visceral neuropathy.

IV. CONCLUSIONS

The use of Holter monitoring to document silent myocardial ischemia in patients experiencing both symptomatic and asymptomatic episodes seems well established. Still uncertain, however, is whether ST changes seen in otherwise healthy individuals (who have not undergone coronary arteriography) has the same connotation. Consequently, the role of routine Holter monitoring in detecting coronary artery disease in a totally asymptomatic population remains unclear. What has become clear, however, is an emerging consensus for what constitutes an ischemic episode on the Holter recording: ST segment depression of at least 1.0 mm (0.1 mV) lasting 1 min and separated from other episodes by at least 1 min [33]. This "1 × 1 × 1" rule should serve as a helpful guideline in defining myocardial ischemia on Holter monitoring. It is also apparent that 24 hours is not the optimum time period for monitoring events; 48 hr seems more appropriate.

REFERENCES

1. H. V. Pipberg, R. C. Arzbaecher, A. S. Berson, S. A. Briller, D. A. Brody, N. C. Flowers, D. B. Geselowitz, E. Lepeschkin, C. G. Oliver, O. H. Schmitt, and M. Spach. Recommendations for standardization of leads and of specifications for instruments in electrocardiography and vectorcardiography: Report of the Committee on Electrocardiography, American Heart Association. *Circulation, 52*:11 (1975).

2. A. Gallino, S. Chierchia, G. Smith, M. Croom, M. Morgan, C. Marchesi, and A. Maseri. Computer system for analysis of ST segment changes on 24 hour Holter monitor tapes: Comparison with other available systems. *J. Am. Coll. Cardiol., 4*:245 (1984).

3. C. R. Lambert, G. A. Imperi, and C. J. Pepine. Low-frequency requirements for recording ischemic ST-segment abnormalities in coronary artery disease. *Am. J. Cardiol., 58*:225 (1986).

4. T. L. Shook, W. Balke, P. W. Kotilainen, M. Hubelbank, A. P. Selwyn, and P. H. Stone. Comparison of amplitude-modulated (direct) and frequency-modulated ambulatory techniques for recording ischemic electrocardiographic changes. *Am. J. Cardiol., 60*:895 (1987).

5. H. L. Kennedy and R. D. Wiens. Ambulatory (Holter) electrocardiography using real-time analysis. *Am. J. Cardiol., 59*:1190 (1987).

6. S. M. Jamal, L. Mitra-Duncan, D. T. Kelly, and S. B. Breedman. Validation of a real-time electrocardiographic monitor for detection of myocardial ischemia secondary to coronary artery disease. *Am. J. Cardiol., 60*:525 (1987).

7. J. Barry, S. Campbell, E. G. Nabel, K. Mead, and A. P. Selwyn. Ambulatory monitoring of the digitized electrocardiogram for detection and early warning of transient myocardial ischemia in angina pectoris. *Am. J. Cardiol., 60*:483 (1987).

8. S. Stern and D. Tzivoni. Early detection of silent ischaemic heart disease by 24-hour ECG monitoring during normal daily activity. *Br. Heart J., 36*:481 (1974).

9. S. Stern and D. Tzivoni. Dynamic changes in the ST-T segment during sleep in ischemic heart disease. *Am. J. Cardiol., 32*:17 (1973).

10. S. Stern, D. Tzivoni, and Z. Stern. Diagnostic accuracy of ambulatory ECG monitoring in ischemic heart disease. *Circulation, 52*:1045 (1975).

11. M. H. Crawford, C. A. Mendoza, R. A. O'Rourke, D. H. White, C. A. Boucher, and J. Gorwit. Limitations of continuous ambulatory electrocardiogram monitoring for detecting coronary artery disease. *Ann. Intern. Med., 89*:1 (1978).

12. S. J. Schang and C. J. Pepine. Transient asymptomatic S-T segment depression during daily activity. *Am. J. Cardiol., 39*:396 (1977).

13. J. E. Deanfield, A. Maseri, A. P. Selwyn, S. Chierchia, P. Ribiero, S. Krikler, and M. Morgan. Myocardial ischemia during daily life in patients with stable angina: Its relation to symptoms and heart rate changes. *Lancet, 2*:753 (1983).

14. J. E. Deanfield, M. Shea, P. Ribiero, C. M. deLandsheere, R. A. Wilson, P. Horlock, and A. P. Selwyn. Transient ST segment depression as a marker of myocardial ischemia during daily life. *Am. J. Cardiol., 54*:1195 (1984).

15. A. C. Cecchi, E. V. Dovellini, F. Marchi, P. Pucci, C. M. Santoro, and P. F. Fazzini. Silent myocardial ischemia during ambulatory electrocardiographic monitoring in patients with effort angina. *J. Am. Coll. Cardiol., 1*:934 (1983).

16. S. H. Kunkes, A. D. Prichard, H. Smith, Jr., R. Gorlin, M. V. Herman, and J. Kupersmith. Silent ST segment deviations and extent of coronary artery disease. *Am. Heart J., 100*:813 (1980).

17. T. vonArnim, B. Hofling, and M. Schreiber. Characteristics of episodes of ST elevation or ST depression during ambulatory monitoring in patients subsequently undergoing coronary angiography. *Br. Heart J., 54*:484 (1985).

18. M. B. Rocco, J. Barry, S. Campbell, E. Nabel, E. F. Cook, L. Goldman, and A. P. Selwyn. Circadian variation of transient myocardial ischemia in patients with coronary artery disease. *Circulation, 75*:395 (1987).

19. D. A. Brezinski, G. H. Tofler, J. E. Muller, S. Pohjola-Sintonen, S. N. Willich, A. I. Schafer, C. A. Czeisler, and G. H. Williams. Morning increase in platelet aggregability: Association with assumption of the upright posture. *Circulation, 78*:35 (1988).

20. S. O. Gottlieb, M. L. Weisfeldt, P. Ouyang, E. D. Mellits, and G. Gerstenblith. Silent ischemia as a marker for early unfavorable outcomes in patients with unstable angina. *N. Engl. J. Med., 314*:1214 (1986).

21. M. A. Josephson, K. Nademanee, V. Intarachot, H. S. Lewis, and B. N. Singh. Abolition of Holter-detected silent myocardial ischemia following percutaneous transluminal coronary angioplasty. *J. Am. Coll. Cardiol., 10*: 499 (1987).

22. D. Tzivoni, A. Gavish, J. Benhorin, S. Banai, A. Keren, and S. Stern. Day-to-day variability of myocardial ischemic episodes in coronary artery disease. *Am. J. Cardiol., 60*:1003 (1987).

23. E. G. Nabel, J. Barry, M. B. Rocco, S. Campbell, K. Mead, T. Fenton, E. J. Orav, and A. P. Selwyn. Variability of transient myocardial ischemia in ambulatory patients with coronary artery disease. *Circulation, 78*:60 (1988).

24. P. F. Cohn, G. W. Vetrovec, R. Nesto, and the Total Ischemia Awareness Program Investigators. A national survey of painful and painless myocardial ischemia: The Total Awareness Program (preliminary report) (abstr). *J. Am. Coll. Cardiol., 11*:203A (1988).

25. W. F. Armstrong and S. N. Morris. The ST segment during ambulatory electrocardiographic monitoring. *Ann. Intern. Med., 98*:249 (1983).

26. A. A. Quyumi, C. Wright, and K. Fox. Ambulatory electrocardiographic ST segment changes in healthy volunteers. *Br. Heart J., 50*:460 (1983).

27. R. S. Kohli, P. M. M. Cashman, A. Lahiri, and E. B. Raftery. The ST segment of the ambulatory electrocardiogram in a normal population. *Br. Heart J. 60*:4 (1988).

28. J. E. Deanfield, P. Ribiero, K. Oakley, S. Krikler, and A. P. Selwyn. Analysis of ST segment changes in normal subjects: Implications for ambulatory monitoring in angina pectoris. *Am. J. Cardiol., 54*:1321 (1984).

29. S. Campbell, J. Barry, G. S. Rebecca, M. B. Rocco, E. G. Nabel, R. R. Wayne, and A. P. Selwyn. Active transient myocardial ischemia during daily life in asymptomatic patients with positive exercise tests and coronary artery disease. *Am. J. Cardiol., 57*:1010 (1986).

30. K. M. Coy, G. A. Imperi, C. R. Lambert, and C. J. Pepine. Silent myocardial ischemia during daily activities in asymptomatic men with positive exercise test responses. *Am. J. Cardiol., 59*:45 (1987).

31. P. F. Cohn and W. E. Lawson. Characteristics of silent myocardial ischemia during out-of-hospital activities in asymptomatic angiographically documented coronary artery disease. *Am. J. Cardiol., 59*:746 (1987).

32. M. Chairiello, C. Indolfi, M. R. Cotecchia, C. Sifola, M. Romano, and M. Condorelli. Asymptomatic transient ST changes during ambulatory ECG monitoring in diabetic patients. *Am. Heart J., 110*:529 (1985).

33. P. F. Cohn and W. B. Kannel (eds.). Recognition, pathogenesis, and management options in silent coronary artery disease. *Circulation, 75*(Suppl II): 1-54 (1987).

9

Exercise Testing

While the Holter monitor is being used with increasing frequency to evaluate silent myocardial ischemia, it still must share center stage with the exercise test. The latter is an established procedure for assessing ischemic responses, arrhythmias and cardiac performance in persons with known or suspected heart disease. In addition, many epidemiologic studies have been performed to evaluate the accuracy of exercise electrocardiographic testing in predicting the occurrence of overt cardiac events in asymptomatic populations. The exercise test has also been used as a procedure to screen asymptomatic individuals in order to identify those persons who

123

warrant further non-invasive or invasive testing because of an abnormal exercise response. The latter approach considers the exercise electrocardiogram as an *indicator* of myocardial ischemia, rather than as only a risk factor for the development of coronary artery disease.

I. EXERCISE TESTS AS PREDICTORS OF FUTURE CARDIAC EVENTS

One of the earliest and largest of the epidemiologic studies was that initiated in 1971 by Bruce and colleagues (the Seattle Heart Watch Study). In this prospective community study of symptom-limited maximal exercise testing, more than 4000 persons clinically free of heart disease were registered between 1971 and 1974. Annual follow-up surveillance of subsequent primary coronary artery disease (defined as admission to a hospital for evaluation or treatment) was continued until the beginning of 1981. A 1983 report [1] provides a unique 10-year experience for evaluating the interactive value of exercise test predictors combined with the usual coronary risk factors (hypertension, hyperlipidemia, diabetes, cigarette smoking) and a family history of premature coronary artery disease, in the 3611 men and 547 women enrolled in this study. Mean age of the men was 45.5 ± 8.4 (SD) years; for the women it was 49.1 ± 9.0 years. The standard Bruce protocol for symptom-limited maximal exercise, using progressive increments in speed and gradient on a motor-driven treadmill, was employed. The most common cause for stopping the tests was fatigue. Patients were divided into subgroups based on presence of conventional risk factors and four abnormal exercise predictors. These included (1) chest pain during the test; (2) inability to complete stage 2 of the protocol; (3) maximal heart rate less than 90% of age-predicted normal value (based on the formulae $y = 227 - 1.067$ [age in years for men] and $y = 206 - 0.597$ [age in years for women]); and (4) development of 1mm or more of horizontal or downsloping ST depression for at least 1 min into the recovery period. Event rates for cardiac events per 1000 person-years of follow-up were calculated. Prior to applying the results of exercise testing, the annual incidence rate of total cardiac events was 0.35% in asymptomatic healthy men and 0.31% in women. When the interaction of any conventional risk factor and two or more of the exercise predictors was considered, the annual risk of cardiac death (for men and women combined) increased from 0.12 % to 9.61% ($p < 0.05$). Six-year survival rates decreased from $97.8 \pm 0.4\%$ to 75.7 ± 7.1 ($p < 0.001$) in this subgroup when life-table analysis was performed (Figure 1).

Other studies have used ST segment depression alone as a predictor of future cardiac events. For example, Ellestad and Wan [2] collected follow-up

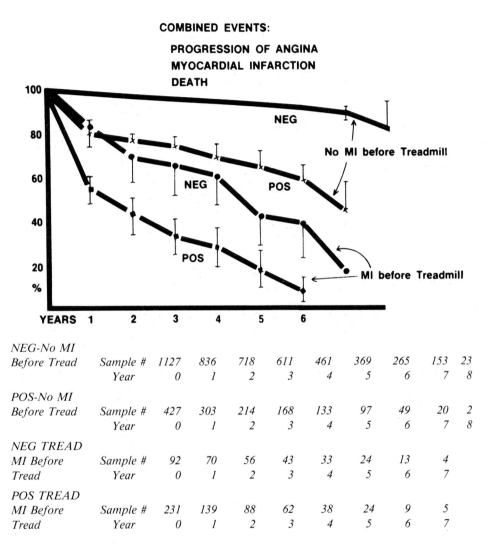

NEG-No MI										
Before Tread	*Sample #*	*1127*	*836*	*718*	*611*	*461*	*369*	*265*	*153*	*23*
	Year	*0*	*1*	*2*	*3*	*4*	*5*	*6*	*7*	*8*
POS-No MI										
Before Tread	*Sample #*	*427*	*303*	*214*	*168*	*133*	*97*	*49*	*20*	*2*
	Year	*0*	*1*	*2*	*3*	*4*	*5*	*6*	*7*	*8*
NEG TREAD										
MI Before	*Sample #*	*92*	*70*	*56*	*43*	*33*	*24*	*13*	*4*	
Tread	*Year*	*0*	*1*	*2*	*3*	*4*	*5*	*6*	*7*	
POS TREAD										
MI Before	*Sample #*	*231*	*139*	*88*	*62*	*38*	*24*	*9*	*5*	
Tread	*Year*	*0*	*1*	*2*	*3*	*4*	*5*	*6*	*7*	

Figure 2   The incidence of all coronary events in the negative and positive ST responders who had not had a previous infarction is compared with the negative and positive responders who had a previous myocardial infarction. (From M. H. Ellestad and M. K. C. Wan. *Circulation, 51*:363, 1975, with permission from the American Heart Association.)

The incidence of coronary events was very low in the controls (0.8% for the first 5 years) as compared to 10.37% in the study group (Figure 2). This difference was higher than that observed in the second five years. Although, as expected, the conventional risk factors were also prognostic indicators in this study, the authors concluded that the positive exercise electrocardiogram was an *independent* risk predictor. In a subsequent letter to the editor of the *New Journal of Medicine* [5], these results were criticized on a cost-benefit basis since it required exercise testing in over 10,000 healthy individuals to produce 135 persons (1.2%) with a positive test, of whom only 21 or (19%) had coronary events over a 5-year period. In their reply, Giagnoni et al. drew attention to the fact that they were not advocating mass screening but rather suggested confining exercise

Table 3 Number and Rate of Coronary Heart Disease Deaths (per 1,000 person-years of risk), Crude Relative Risk and Cox Adjusted Relative Risk[a] by the Presence of Exercise Electrocardiographic Abnormalities for Multiple Risk Factor Intervention Trial Usual Care Men

	Exercise ECG				Relative risk	Cox adjusted relative risk
	Normal		Abnormal			
End point	No.	Rate/1000	No.	Rate/1000		
CHD death	73	2.0	38	7.61	3.80**	3.45*
CVD death	90	2.48	40	8.02	3.25**	2.99**
Non-CVD death	101	2.78	5	1.00	0.36*	0.35*
All deaths	191	5.25	45	9.02	1.72**	1.61**
Angina	632	18.34	132	28.26	1.55**	1.58**
Nonfatal MI by serial ECG change	129	3.53	18	3.54	1.04	0.93
Definite clinical MI	183	5.03	31	6.21	1.25	1.17
CHD death, serial ECG change or definite clinical MI	356	9.79	85	17.04	1.76**	1.67**

*$p < 0.05$.
**$p < 0.01$.
[a]Adjusted for age, diastolic pressure, serum cholesterol and number of cigarettes smoked daily.
CHD = coronary heart disease; CVD = cardiovascular disease; ECG = electrocardiogram; MI = myocardial infarction.
Source: P. M. Rautaharju, R. J. Prineas, W. J. Eifler, C. D. Furberg, J. F. Neaton, R. S. Crow, J. Stamler, and J. A. Cutler. *J. Am. Coll. Cardiol.*, 8:1, 1986.

testing to males over 45 with "high levels" of conventional risk factors. This is also my approach. The two most recent studies of this type are the MRFIT study [6] and the Lipid Research Clinics Mortality Follow-Up Study [7]. In the former, involving over 6000 men, a positive exercise test was associated with nearly a fourfold (3.80) risk of death for coronary heart disease (Table 3) during a 7-year follow-up period. In the latter,

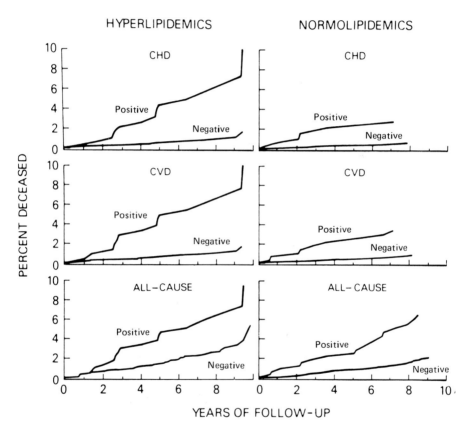

Figure 3 Age-adjusted life table curves for men with positive and negative exercise tests within the hyperlipidemic (left) and normolipidemic (right) subpopulations. These six pairs of curves were generated from six separate proportional-hazards models, each containing age as a continuous variable and exercise test outcome as a categorical variable. (From D. J. Gordon, L-G. Ekelund, J. M. Karon, J. L. Probstfiedl, C. Rubeinstein, L. T. Sheffield, and L. Weissfeld. *Circulation, 74*:252, 1986.)

involving over 3000 men, a positive exercise test was associated with a cumulative mortality of 11.9% over 8.1 years mean follow-up time, versus 1.2% over 8.6 years for men with a negative test. This occurred despite similar levels of serum cholesterol in both groups (Figure 3). In contrast to these studies, McHenry et al. [8] have reported that ST segment depression predicts an increased incidence of angina as the initial coronary event, but not infarction or death.

Exercise-induced ventricular premature beats, as opposed to ST segment depression or duration of exercise, do not appear to be reliable predictors of cardiac events in asymptomatic persons.

II. EXERCISE TESTS AS INDICATORS OF ASYMPTOMATIC CORONARY ARTERY DISEASE

In my opinion, what is overlooked in the epidemiologic studies cited is that the abnormal ST segment response may be more than merely a risk factor that *predicts* disease. An abnormal response may instead by an *indicator* that latent disease is already present. To confirm this hypothesis, it would be necessary to submit positive responders to coronary arteriography, i.e., "case finding." However, the frequency of false-positive responses in an asymptomatic population is high, based on low disease prevalence, i.e., Bayes' theorem (9), discussed at length in Chapter 10. For example, Erikssen et al. [10], in their studies of Norwegian factory workers, selected 115 men out of a cohort of 2014 presumably healthy men based on a positive exercise test. Of the 115, 105 underwent coronary angiography but only 69 had significant disease (75% stenosis). In Froelicher's study of U.S. Air Force personnel [11], 1390 men were exercised and 135 had abnormal tests. Only 35 (25.4%) had significant coronary artery disease. When Hopkirk et al. [12] added more study subjects to Froelicher's original group and then investigated the predictive value of exercise duration plus persistence of ST depression plus the depth of ST depression, they achieved almost 90% predictive accuracy for coronary artery disease, and a predictive value only slightly less than that for multi-vessel disease (84%). The three test variables (i.e., those with the highest "likelihood ratio") were 3 mm or more of ST segment depression, persistence of ST depression 5 min after exercise, and total duration of exercise of less than 10 min. The combination of any two of these three exercise risk predictors plus one of the conventional risk factors yielded the predictive value noted earlier.

Other investigators [13-15] have also examined the degree of ST depression and its persistence into the recovery period with or without hypotension. They agree that the greater the ischemic change, the more likely asymptomatic or minimally symptomatic patients will have severe disease. For example, in the study by Hamby et al. [15] (Table 4), 27 patients had positive exercise tests. Of the six with an abnormal blood pressure response, five (or 83%) had left main or triple-vessel disease. By contrast, only 9 of the 21 persons (43%) with a normal blood pressure response had this finding on coronary angiography.

Changes in the R wave on the electrocardiogram have also been looked at specifically in studies of U.S. Air Force personnel; 65 men with coronary artery disease and 190 normal subjects formed the study population [16] (Table 5). R-wave amplitude changes were evaluated in bipolar leads X, Y and Z. Exercise-induced changes in R-wave height (diminution or no change) increased the specificity of detecting coronary artery disease in asymptomatic men over ST segment criteria alone, but the sensitivity was poor and the overall predictive value not enhanced. These results differ from those of Yiannikas et al. [17], who have found that the R wave response was more helpful than ST segment responses. As noted earlier, Allen et al. [3] also used the R wave response in combination with other ECG measurements to improve diagnostic accuracy in asymptomatic men.

Table 4 Relation of Exercise Blood Pressure Response to Main Left or Triple-Vessel Coronary Disease, or Both

	Patient group			
	A (n = 27)	B (n = 36)	C (n = 57)	Total (n = 120)
Abnormal blood pressure response	6	9	21	36[a]
Left main or triple vessel coronary disease (%)	5 (83%)	8 (89%[a])	17 (81%)	30 (83%)
Normal blood pressure response	21	27	36	84[a]
Main left or triple vessel coronary disease, or both (%)	9 (43%)	8 (30%[a])	25 (69%)	42 (50%)

[a] $p < 0.01$ (comparison of percent of patients in group B with left main or triple vessel coronary disease, or both, in the subgroups with abnormal and normal blood pressure responses).
Group A = no angina; Group B = mild angina; Group C = moderate angina.
Source: R. I. Hamby, E. T. Davison, J. Hilsenrath, S. Shanies, M. Young, D. H. Murphy, and I. Hoffman. *J. Am. Coll. Cardiol., 3*:1375, 1984.

Table 5 Diagnostic Accuracy of Different Criteria in Detecting Different Angiographic Definitions of Coronary Artery Disease (50 or 70% Reduction [R] in Luminal Diameter or Multivessel Disease [MVD])[a]

	Sensitivity (%)			Specificity (%)			Predictive Value (%)		
	50 R	70 R	MVD	50 R	70 R	MVD	50 R	70 R	MVD
ST depression	—	—	—	—	—	—	25	18	14
R wave amplitude at stress									
↑ X	28	28	31	87	86	86	42	30	28
↑ Y	32	33	32	81	80	81	37	26	32
↑ ΣXY	22	24	26	88	88	88	38	30	34
↓ Z	82	97	95	20	5	16	26	2	16

[a]Multivessel disease = coronary disease, defined as 50% reduction of luminal diameter, in two or three major vessels. ↑ = increase; ↓ = decrease. X, Y and Z refer to X, Y and Z bipolar leads. *Source*: J. A. C. Hopkirk, C. S. Uhl, J. R. Hickman, Jr., and J. Fischer. *J. Am. Coll. Cardiol., 3*: 821, 1984.

There are two other settings in which exercise test results are of importance. The first is in detecting silent coronary artery disease in diabetic populations [18,19], and the second is in combination with Holter monitoring. In the latter instance, the exercise test can be used to "calibrate" the Holter [20] and to indicate which patients are most likely to develop out-of-hospital ischemic events [21], i.e., those with exercise induced ischemia at less than 6 min of exercise duration (Figure 4). Prognostic risk stratification is also enhanced when both procedures are combined (see Chapter 12).

III. CONCLUSIONS

Abnormal exercise test responses in asymptomatic populations not only appear to be reliable *predictors* of future cardiac events, but they also are valuable as *indicators* of occult coronary artery disease. Because of the problem of false-positive responses in an asymptomatic population, stress tests should be considered as screening procedures for coronary artery disease only in those individuals with multiple risk factors and/or family histories of premature coronary artery disease. The abnormal test is more likely to be a "true-positive" response when other abnormalities besides ST changes are present.

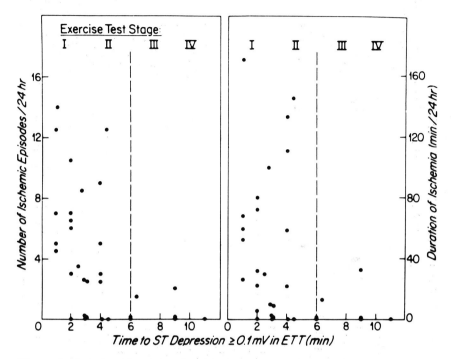

Figure 4 Relationship of time in minutes to onset of significant ST depression (≥0.1 mV) during the Bruce protocol exercise test to degree of ischemic activity out of hospital as detected by ambulatory monitoring, expressed as number of ischemic episodes per 24 hr (left) and total duration of ischemia in minutes per 24 hr (right) in patients with electrocardiographically positive exercise tests (group I). Stages of the Bruce protocol are listed at the top of each panel. Note that the frequency and duration of ischemia out of hospital declines as the time to ischemia during exercise increases, especially after 6 or more min (end of stage II). (From S. Campbell, J. Barry, M. B. Rocco, E. G. Nable, K. Mead-Walters, G. S. Rebecca, and A. P. Selwyn. *Circulation, 74*:72, 1986.)

REFERENCES

1. R. A. Bruce, K. F. Hossack, T. A. DeRouen, and V. Hofer. Enhanced risk assessment for primary coronary heart disease events by maximal exercise testing: 10 years' experience of Seattle Heart Watch. *J. Am. Coll. Cardiol., 2*:565 (1983).

2. M. H. Ellestad and M. K. C. Wan. Predictive implications of stress testing: Follow-up of 2700 subjects after maximum treadmill stress testing. *Circulation, 51*:363 (1975).

3. W. H. Allen, S. W. Aronow, P. Goodman, and P. Stinson. Five-year follow-up of maximal treadmill stress test in asymptomatic men and women. *Circulation, 62*:522 (1980).

4. E. Giagnoni, M. B. Secchi, S. C. Wu, A. Morabito, L. Oltrona, S. Mancarella, N. Volpin, L. Fossa, L. Bettazzi, G. Arangio, A. Sachero, and G. Folli. Prognostic value of exercise EKG testing in asymptomatic normotensive subjects: A prospective matched study. *N. Engl. J. Med., 309*:1085 (1983).

5. D. Nicklin and D. J. Balaban. Exercise EKG in asymptomatic normotensive subjects. *N. Engl. J. Med., 310*:853 (1984).

6. P. M. Rautaharju, R. J. Prineas, W. J. Eifler, C. D. Furberg, J. D. Neaton, R. S. Crow, J. Stamler, and J. S. Cutler. Prognostic value of exercise electrocardiogram in men at high risk of future coronary heart disease: Multiple Risk Factor Intervention Trial Experience. *J. Am. Coll. Cardiol., 8*:1 (1986).

7. D. J. Gordon, L-G. Elelund, J. M. Karon, J. L. Probstfield, C. Rubenstein, L. T. Sheffield, and L. Weissfeld. Predictive value of the exercise test for mortality in North American men: The Lipid Research Clinics Mortality Follow-Up Study. *Circulation, 2*:252 (1986).

8. P. L. McHenry, J. O'Donnell, S. N. Norris, and J. J. Jordon. The abnormal exercise electrocardiogram in apparently healthy men: A predictor of angina pectoris as an initial coronary event during long-term follow-up. *Circulation, 70*:547 (1984).

9. R. Detrano, J. Yiannikas, E. E. Salcedo, G. Rincon, R. T. Go, G. Williams, and J. Leatherman. Bayesian probability analysis: A prospective demonstration of its clinical utility in diagnosing coronary disease. *Circulation, 69*:541 (1984).

10. J. Erikssen, I. Enge, R. Forfang, and D. Storstein. False positive diagnostic tests of coronary angiographic findings in 105 presumably healthy males. *Circulation, 54*:371 (1976).

11. V. F. Froelicher, A. J. Thompson, M. R. Longo, Jr., J. H. Triebwasser, and M. C. Lancaster. Value of exercise testing for screening asymptomatic men for latent coronary artery disease. *Prog. Cardiovasc. Dis., 18*:265 (1976).

12. J. A. C. Hopkirk, G. S. Uhl, J. R. Hickman, Jr., J. Fischer, and A. Medina. Discriminant value of clinical and exercise variables in detecting significant coronary artery disease in asymptomatic men. *J. Am. Coll. Cardiol., 3*:887 (1984).

13. D. S. Blumental, J. L. Weiss, E. D. Mellits, and G. Gerstenblith. The predictive value of a strongly positive stress test in patients with minimal symptoms. *Am. J. Med., 70*:1005 (1981).

14. E. C. Lozner and J. Morganroth. New criteria to enhance the predictability of coronary artery disease by exercise testing in asymptomatic subjects. *Circulation, 56*:799 (1977).

15. R. I. Hamby, E. T. Dvison, J. Hilsenrath, S. Shanies, M. Young, D. H. Murphy, and I. Hoffman. Functional and anatomic correlates of markedly abnormal stress tests. *J. Am. Coll. Cardiol., 3*:1375 (1984).

16. J. A. C. Hopkirk, G. S. Uhl, J. R. Hickman, Jr., and J. Fischer. Limitation of exercise-induced R wave amplitude changes in detecting coronary artery disease in asymptomatic men. *J. Am. Coll. Cardiol., 3*:821 (1984).

17. J. Yiannikas, J. Marcomichelakis, P. Taggart, B. H. Keely, and R. Emanuel. Analysis of exercise-induced changes in R wave amplitude in asymptomatic men with electrocardiographic ST-T changes at rest. *Am. J. Cardiol., 47*:238 (1981).

18. S. R. Chipkin, D. Frid, J. S. Alpert, S. P. Baker, J. E. Dalen, and N. Aronin. Frequency of painless myocardial ischemia during exercise tolerance testing in patients with and without diabetes mellitus. *Am. J. Cardiol., 59*:61 (1987).

19. S. Rubler, D. Gerber, J. Reitano, V. Chokshi, and V. J. Fisher. Predictive value of clinical and exercise variables for detection of coronary artery disease in men with diabetes mellitus. *Am. J. Cardiol., 59*:1310 (1987).

20. D. Tzivoni, J. Benhorin, A. Gavish, and S. Stern. Holter recording during treadmill testing in assessing myocardial ischemic changes. *Am. J. Cardiol., 55*:1200 (1985).

21. S. Campbell, J. Barry, M. B. Rocco, E. G. Nabel, K. Mead-Walters, G. S. Rebecca, and A. P. Selwyn. Features of the exercise test that reflect the activity of ischemic heart disease out of hospital. *Circulation, 1*:72 (1986).

10
Combining the Exercise Test with Other Procedures

In patients with angina or prior myocardial infarctions, the positive but painless exercise test can often stand alone as a true marker of silent ischemia. But this is not true in asymptomatic populations. There, we usually combine the exercise test with other procedures in order to increase the reliability of detecting occult coronary artery disease. This is necessary because of the frequency of false-positive test responses, which is a function of Bayes' theorem. This theorem was alluded to in the preceding chapter but several points deserve further emphasis.

I. BAYES' THEOREM

Bayes' theorem states that test results cannot be adequately interpreted without knowing the prevalence of the disease in the population under study. This is called the pretest likelihood (or prior probability) of disease, as opposed to the posttest likelihood (or posterior probability). Definitions and equations for these terms are as follows:

Pretest likelihood (*prior probability*) is defined as the probability of disease in a subject to be tested

$$= \frac{\text{number of patients with disease in the test population}}{\text{total number of patients in the test population}} \tag{1}$$

Posttest likelihood (*posterior probability*) is defined as the probability of disease in a subject showing a given test result

$$= \frac{\text{number of patients with disease showing a given test result}}{\text{total number of subjects showing the test result}} \tag{2}$$

Bayes' theorem helps to explain the well-known observation that a small proportion of normal persons will have a "false-positive" response; i.e., they will have an abnormal test response but will prove to be normal on more exact study. A good example is an abnormal exercise test response that is suggestive of coronary artery disease in a person who subsequently undergoes coronary angiography and is found to have normal coronary arteries. In short, the predictive value of any less-than-perfect test, such as the exercise stress test, is reduced to an extent that is related in part to the fraction of normal persons in the study population [1].

Epstein [2] gives two examples to illustrate this point. Key terms are sensitivity, specificity and predictive value. These are defined as follows with appropriate equations also provided:

Sensitivity is defined as the probability a patient with disease will have a given test result

$$= \frac{\text{number of patients with disease with a given test result}}{\text{total number of diseased subjects tested}} \tag{3}$$

Specificity is defined as the probability a patient with disease will have a given test result

$$= \frac{\text{number of patients without disease without a given test result}}{\text{total number of disease-free subjects tested}} \tag{4}$$

Predictive value of a positive test is defined as the probability that a patient has disease, given a positive test outcome

$$= \frac{\text{number of patients with disease}}{\text{total number of patients with a positive test}} \qquad (5)$$

Predictive value of a negative test is defined as the probability that a patient does not have disease, given a negative test outcome

$$= \frac{\text{number of subjects without disease}}{\text{total number of subjects with a negative test}} \qquad (6)$$

Assuming exercise tests have a sensitivity of 75% and a specificity of 85%, what are the chances that a positive test in any *asymptomatic* per-

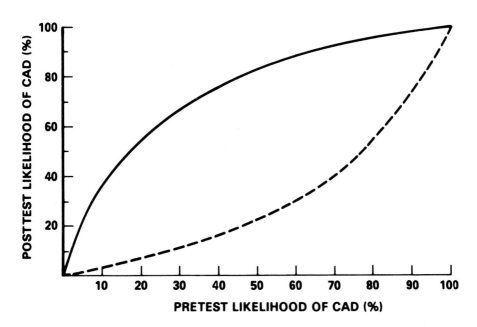

Figure 1 Influence of pretest likelihood of coronary artery disease (CAD) on the posttest likelihood of coronary artery disease. _____ = positive test (sensitivity 75%); - - - = negative test (specificity 85%). (From S. E. Epstein, *Am. J. Cardiol., 46*:491, 1980.)

son (with a 3% pretest likelihood of coronary artery disease) truly indicates coronary artery disease? The answer is that the positive test's predictive value (or posttest likelihood) of disease being present is 14%. By contrast, the same positive test result in a person *with angina* (and thus a 90% pretest likelihood of coronary artery disease) yields a 98% posttest likelihood. The predictive value of a negative test is inverse to that of a positive test. The complete spectrum of pre- and posttest likelihoods of the exercise test predicting coronary artery disease is depicted in Figure 1. The posttest likelihoods are highest in those individuals with a high pretest likelihood and vice versa. The low predictive value in asymptomatic subjects has led investigators to search for other ways of increasing the posttest likelihood. One way is to construct a "family" of ST segment depression curves as in Figure 2. We now no longer look upon the exercise test as merely providing a "yes or no" statement regarding the presence of coronary artery disease, but as providing a continuum of risk based on different probability estimates. A "very positive" test, i.e., one with more than 2.5 mm of ST depression, greatly increases the posttest likelihood of coronary artery disease.

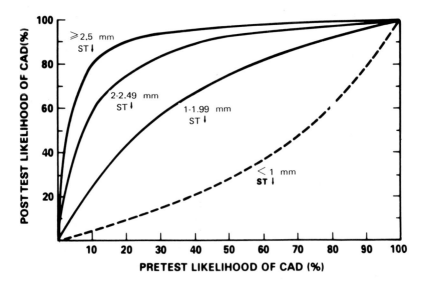

Figure 2   Family of ST segment depression curves (based on data derived from Diamond and Forrester [3] and likelihood of coronary artery disease (CAD). ST↓ segment depression. (From S. E. Epstein, *Am. J. Cardiol.*, *46*:491, 1980.)

II. ADDING OTHER PROCEDURES INCREASES POSTTEST LIKELIHOOD

When *conventional risk factors* are taken into consideration, a high-risk subgroup can be identified in which a positive exercise test has more validity than in a low-risk group. Several groups have used data from the *Coronary Risk Handbook* based on the Framingham Study to provide relevant data. As seen in Figure 3, a 55-year-old man with a cholesterol

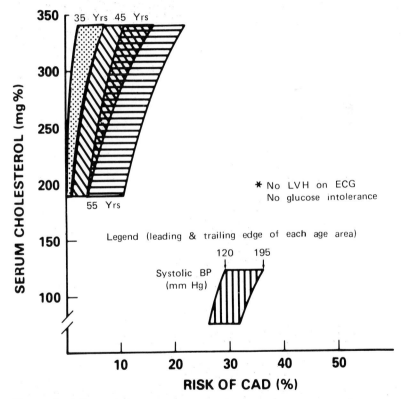

Figure 3 Effect of age, serum cholesterol and blood pressure (BP) on risk of coronary artery disease (CAD) in nonsmoking men 35 to 55 years of age. (The graph is based on data derived from the Framingham Study, in which the cholesterol values were obtained using the Abell-Kendall method. Most direct and automated cholesterol determinations give values 5-15% above that given in this graph). ECG = electrocardiogram; LVH = left ventricular hypertrophy. (From S. E. Epstein. *Am. J. Cardiol., 46*:491, 1980.)

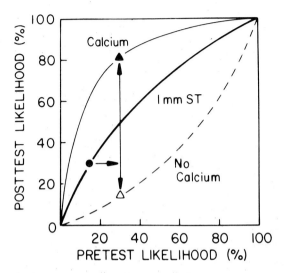

Figure 4 Influence of serial tests on posttest likelihood. The closed circle represents a patient with a pretest likelihood of 15% (X axis) and a 1.0-mm depression of the ST segment after a stress test (heavy solid line). The resultant posttest likelihood is 27% (Y axis). If cardiac fluoroscopy showed calcification of one coronary vessel (light solid line), the resultant posttest likelihood would rise (↑) to 79% (▲). If no calcification was observed (dashed line), the likelihood would fall (↓) to 14% (△). Note that the posttest likelihood from the first test becomes the pretest likelihood of the second test (horizontal arrow). (From G. A. Diamond and J. S. Forrester. *N. Engl. J. Med., 300*:1350, 1979.)

level of 350 mg% and a systolic blood pressure of 195 mmHg would have a 20% pretest risk of coronary artery disease. With a positive exercise test, posttest likelihood could increase to 50-90% depending on the degree of ST segment depression.

When a second independent test is employed, the posttest likelihood from the exercise test becomes the pretest likelihood for the second test. An example is the demonstration of *coronary artery calcification* by fluoroscopy, as depicted by Diamond and Forrester [3] in Figure 4. This particular observation is based partly on the work of Langou et al. [4], who have shown that the presence of coronary artery calcification is a powerful predictor of coronary artery disease in asymptomatic men with a positive exercise test. Langou et al. [4] screened 120 middle-aged males free of clinical heart disease. Of the original group, 108 completed the submaximal exercise protocol by achieving at least 90% of their age-predicted maximal heart rate; these subjects made up the study population. Sixteen subjects had a positive exercise test; 13 (81%) also had at least one calcified artery on fluoroscopy. By contrast, only 13 (35%) of the 37 subjects with coronary artery calcification had a positive exercise test. Cardiac catheterization was performed in the 13 men with both a positive exercise test and coronary calcification. As depicted in Table 1, one subject had <50% luminal stenosis; all the rest had at least 75% luminal stenosis in one vessel with five persons having two-vessel disease and three having three-vessel disease. Thus, the predictive accuracy obtained by combining both noninvasive tests was 92%.

The influence of other serial tests besides cardiac fluoroscopy on post-test likelihood has also been studied. Diamond et al. [5] evaluated other noninvasive tests including the stress cardiokymograph, which is used for the detection of precordial regional left ventricular dysfunction (noted previously in Chapter 7), and stress thallium-201 scintigraphy for assessment of exercise-induced regional myocardial hypoperfusion. The greater the number of abnormal responses observed in a given patient, the greater the predictive accuracy for coronary artery disease and especially multivessel disease. Of the 974 patients studied in this manner, 278 (29%) were asymptomatic. A computer-assisted program (called CADENZA) was used to analyze and report the results of the various tests (Table 2).

Epstein [2] also considered serial testing with *radionuclide procedures* since they have a higher predictive value than the exercise ECG alone. He reasoned that the combination of a positive exercise ECG and either an abnormal thallium perfusion scan or radionuclide ventriculogram would markedly increase the predictive value of the exercise test (Figure 5), although he cautioned that sensitivity and specificity of these tests in asymptomatic persons might well be different from that in symptomatic patients.

Table 1 Predictive Accuracy of Coronary Artery Calcification at Fluoroscopy and Abnormal Exercise Stress Test

	No. pts.	Significant CAD	CAD
Coronary calcification			
+			
abnormal exercise test	13	12	13
Predictive accuracy		92%	100%

Source: R. A. Langou, E. K. Huang, M. J. Kelley, and L. S. Cohen. *Circulation, 62*:1196, 1980.

Table 2 Variables Analyzed by CADENZA

Variable	Measurement interval	Conditional variable
History		
Age (yr)	Continuous	—
Sex	Male. female	—
Chest discomfort	AS. NA. AA. TA	Age. sex
Systolic BP (mm Hg)	Continuous	Sex
Cholesterol (mg/dl)	Continuous	Age. sex
Currently smoking	Yes. no	Sex
Glucose intolerance	Yes. no	Sex
Rest ECG	Normal. abnormal	Sex
ECG stress test		
Duration of exercise (min)	Continuous	—
Magnitude of ST depression (mm)	< 0.5. 0.5. 1.0. 1.5. 2.0. > 2.5	Sex. rest ECG
Slope of ST segment	Upsloping. horizontal. down-sloping	Rest ECG
R wve amplitude change (mm)	Continuous	—
Fluoroscopy		
No. of calcified vessels	0. 1. 2. 3	Age
Cardiokymography		
Rest pattern	I. II. III.	—
Postexercise pattern	I. II. III	Rest pattern
Thallium scintigraphy		
Type of defect	None, fixed, reversible	—
Magnitude of defect	Mild, moderate, severe	Type of defect
Pulmonary uptake	None, mild/moderate, moderate/severe	—
Technetium scintigraphy		
Rest ejection fraction (%)	Continuous	—
Peak exercise ejection fraction (%)	Continuous	—

AA = atypical angina; AS = asymptomatic; BP = blood pressure; ECG = electrocardiogram; I = inward systolic motion; II = mid-systolic outward motion; III = holosystolic outward motion; NA = nonanginal discomfort; TA = typical angina.
Source: G. A. Diamond, H. M. Staniloff, J. S. Forrester, B. H. Pollack, and H. J. C. Swan. *J. Am. Coll. Cardiol., 1*:444, 1983.

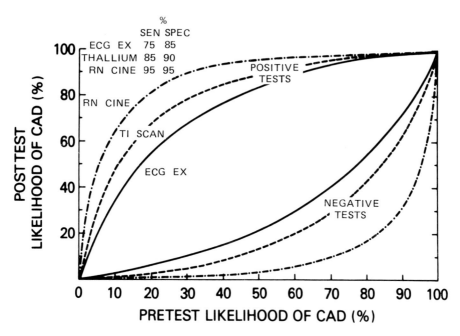

Figure 5   Probability of coronary artery disease (CAD). Comparison of electrocardiographic exercise testing (ECG EX), thallium perfusion scanning (TI SCAN)
and radionuclide cineangiography (RN CINE). (Sensitivity [SEN] and specificity
[SPEC] values are approximations derived from published series.) (From S. E.
Epstein. *Am. J. Cardiol., 46*:491, 1980.)

(In his most recent communication, he continues to be cautious about the
value of screening protocols in asymptomatic populations [6].) The attrac-
tiveness of the radionuclide procedures has been reviewed by Rozanski
and Berman [7] and is based on several studies of asymptomatic persons.
For example, Caralis et al. [8] found that 22 persons out of 3496 developed
2 mm or more ST segment depression on exercise testing. Of the 22 persons, 15 agreed to undergo thallium-201 exercise scintigrams: 10 were abnormal. Nolewaijka et al. [9] found less promising results in their study
of 58 asymptomatic men studied. Of the five men with abnormal thallium
scans, subsequent coronary arteriography in three was normal. Guiney et
al. [10] had similar results in their study of 35 patients. Uhl et al. [11]
studied 191 airmen with abnormal exercise ECGs. Predictive value of the
ECG was 21%, compared to 75% on scintigraphy. They felt the thallium

Table 3 Comparison of Thallium Scintigraphy and Radionuclide Angiography

	Thallium 201		Ejection fraction		Wall motion		Ejection fraction + wall motion
	Normal	Abnormal	Normal	Abnormal	Normal	Abnormal	Abnormal
Normal	18	1	16	3	18	1	1
Coronary artery							
disease	1	12	2	11	5	8	7
Sensitivity	92%		85%		62%		
Specificity	95%		85%		95%		

Source: G. G. Uhl, T. N. Kay, and J. R. Hickman, Jr. *J. Cardiac. Rehabil.*, 2:118, 1982.

test was a good second-line screening procedure. They also compared the thallium-201 myocardial scintigram to the radionuclide ventriculogram; 32 airmen with abnormal exercise ECGs had both thallium scintigrams and radionuclide ventriculograms. Thirteen patients had angiographically documented coronary artery disease; 12 had abnormal thallium scans; 11 had reduced ejection fractions at maximal exercise. Table 3 compares the sensitivity and specificity of the two procedures.

On the basis of these observations, serial testing procedures have been advocated for use in U.S. Air Force personnel, as described by Uhl and Froelicher [12] and recently updated by Schwartz et al. [13]. After initial history, physical examination and resting ECG are performed, a fasting biochemical profile is obtained, and a risk factor index calculated based on Framingham data. Men with positive exercise tests then undergo cardiac fluoroscopy and thallium perfusion scintigraphy before being considered for cardiac catheterization. These authors have stressed the importance of lipid screening, citing the U.S. Air Force studies described in Chapter 7, in which the ratio of total cholesterol to high-density lipoprotein (HDL) cholesterol was a useful predictor of disease. Only 42 (9.5%) of 440 men with abnormal exercise test had a ratio greater than 6.0; by contrast, 87% of those with coronary artery disease had this findings for an odds ratio of 172 to 1 [14]. The U.S. Army also has a similar cardiovascular screening program [15] (Table 4).

At the Johns Hopkins Hospital, serial testing procedures are used to identify high risk subgroups in families with early coronary artery disease. Hypertension and hyperlipidemia in asymptomatic siblings were

Table 4 Criteria for Primary Cardiovascular Screen Failure in the U.S. Army Over-Forty Program[a]

Framingham risk index of 5% or greater
Abnormal cardiovascular history or examination
Electrocardiogram abnormality
(LVH, interventricular conduction defects, ST-T wave changes, etc.)
Fasting blood sugar $\geq$ 115 mg/dl

[a]Any one abnormality requires secondary screening. LVH = left ventricular hypertrophy.
Source: J. M. Zoltick, H. A. McAllister, and J. L. Bedynek, Jr. *J. Cardiac Rehabil.*, *4*:530, 1984.

strongly correlated with positive stress thallium tests. In one subgroup, for example, men over the age of 40 with a systolic blood pressure greater than 150 mmHg had an 82% prevalence of positive stress tests [16]. In this preliminary report, coronary arteriographic findings were not presented, but 2-year follow-up has shown a 6% frequency of subsequent myocardial infarction [17].

As noted in preceeding chapters, diabetic populations show an especially high prevalence of exercise-induced silent ischemia. This is true not only for ECG findings, but also thallium defects [18]. Other studies involving thallium scintigraphy have been reported in asymptomatic post-infarction patients; this avoids problems in interpreting ST depression which may be artificial ("reciprocal changes").

III. CONCLUSIONS

In asymptomatic patients with no prior history of coronary artery disease, noninvasive detection of coronary artery disease is best approached with a variety of procedures that can confirm an abnormal stress test, since the next step—cardiac catheterization—should only be performed when there is a very high suspicion that latent coronary atherosclerosis is present.

REFERENCES

1. R. D. Rifkin and W. B. Hood, Jr. Bayesian analysis of electrocardiographic exercise stress testing. *N. Engl. J. Med.*, *297*:681 (1977).
2. S. E. Epstein. Implications of probability analysis on the strategy used for noninvasive detection of coronary artery disease: Role of single or combined

use of exercise electrocardiographic testing, radionuclide cineangiography and myocardial perfusion imaging. *Am. J. Cardiol., 46*:491 (1980).

3. G. A. Diamond and J. S. Forrester. Analysis of probability as an aid in the clinical diagnosis of coronary artery disease. *N. Engl. J. Med., 300*:1350 (1979).

4. R. A. Langou, E. K. Huang, M. J. Keeley, and L. S. Cohen. Predictive accuracy of coronary artery disease in asymptomatic men. *Circulation, 62*:1196 (1980).

5. G. A. Diamond, H. M. Staniloff, J. S. Forrester, B. H. Pollack, and H. J. C. Swan. Computer-assisted diagnosis in the noninvasive evaluation of patients with suspected coronary artery disease. *J. Am. Coll. Cardiol., 1*:444 (1983).

6. S. E. Epstein, A. A. Quyyumi, and R. O. Bonow. Myocardial ischemia—Silent or symptomatic. *N. Engl. J. Med., 318*:1038 (1988).

7. A. Rozanski and D. S. Berman. Silent myocardial ischemia. I. Pathophysiology, frequency of occurrence, and approaches toward detection. *Am. Heart J., 114*:615 (1987).

8. D. G. Caralis, I. Bailey, H. L. Kennedy, and B. Pitt. Thallium-201 myocardial imaging in evaluation of asymptomatic individuals with ischaemic ST segment depression on exercise electrocardiogram. *Br. Heart J., 42*:452 (1979).

9. A. J. Nolewaijka, W. J. Kostuk, J. Howard, et al. Thallium stress myocardial imaging: An evaluation of fifty-eight asymptomatic males. *Clin. Cardiol., 4*:135 (1981).

10. T. E. Guiney, G. M. Pohost, K. A. McKusick, and G. A. Beller. Differentiation of false- from true-positive ECG responses to exercise stress by thallium-201 perfusion imaging. *Chest, 80*:1 (1981).

11. G. S. Uhl, T. N. Kay, and J. R. Hickman, Jr. Comparison of exercise radionuclide angiography and thallium perfusion imaging in detecting coronary artery disease in asymptomatic men. *J. Cardiac. Rehabil., 2*:118 (1982).

12. G. S. Uhl and V. Froelicher. Screening for asymptomatic coronary artery disease. *J. Am. Coll. Cardiol., 1*:946 (1983).

13. R. S. Schwartz, W. G. Jackson, P. V. Cello, and J. R. Hickman. Exercise thallium-201 scintigraphy for detecting coronary artery disease in asymptomatic young men (abstr). *J. Am. Coll. Cardiol., 11*:80A (1988).

14. G. S. Uhl, R. G. Troxler, J. R. Hickman, Jr., and D. Clark. Relation between high density lipoprotein cholesterol and coronary artery disease in asymptomatic men. *Am. J. Cardiol., 48*:903 (1981).

15. J. M. Zoltick, H. A. McAllister, and J. L. Bedynek, Jr. The United States Army Cardiovascular Screening Program. *J. Cardiac Rehabil., 4*:530 (1984).

16. D. M. Becker, T. Pearson, D. J. Fintel, D. M. Levine, and L. C. Becker. Risk factors identify high risk subgroups in families with early coronary heart disease (CHD). (abstr). *Circulation, 70*(Suppl II):127 (1984).

17. L. C. Becker, D. M. Becker, T. A. Pearson, D. J. Fintel, J. Links, and T. L. Frank. Screening of asymptomatic siblings of patients with premature coronary artery disease. *Circulation, 75*(Suppl II):14, 1987.

18. R. W. Nesto, R. T. Phillips, K. G. Kett, T. Hill, E. Perper, E. Young, and O. S. Leland, Jr. Angina and exertional myocardial ischemia in diabetic and nondiabetic patients: Assessment by exercise thallium scintigraphy. *Ann. Intern. Med., 108*:170 (1988).

11
Cardiac Catheterization

Despite considerable advances in noninvasive imaging technology, cardiac catheterization (including coronary arteriography and usually left ventriculography) is still the accepted standard for the in vivo diagnosis of coronary artery disease. Indications for performing the procedure are still not uniformly agreed upon [1]. Because of this uncertainty, there is considerable controversy when a patient with asymptomatic coronary artery disease is detected via the noninvasive procedures discussed in Chapters 7 through 10, and coronary arteriography is considered to confirm the diagnosis. This controversy is most marked in totally asymptomatic persons and less so in those who are asymptomatic following a myocardial infarction. In those individuals with episodes of both symptomatic and asymptomatic myocardial ischemia, there is the least amount of controversy.

I. INDICATIONS FOR CARDIAC CATHETERIZATION IN TOTALLY ASYMPTOMATIC PERSONS

Ambrose [1] concluded that coronary arteriography "appears warranted in patients with objective evidence of significant ischemia at low work loads even though they are asymptomatic or minimally symptomatic. The purpose of catheterization is to identify those patients with significant coronary artery disease, so that appropriate therapy can be instituted if considered necessary." Before proceeding to catheterization, Ambrose emphasizes the need for a confirmatory radionuclide procedure in addition to a positive exercise test. This is in keeping with Conti's philosophy [2], among others, and it is certainly one that I concur with. The flow diagram that Conti uses to illustrate the subsequent evaluation of asymptomatic patients with a positive exercise test is depicted in Figure 1. In summary, these authors and myself feel that a positive exercise test should be followed by another independent demonstration of ischemia, such as an abnormal thallium-201 scintigram or radionuclide ventriculogram, or demonstration of coronary artery calcification on fluoroscopy before proceeding to cardiac catheterization, an invasive procedure with small but definite associated morbidity and mortality.

Of course, not all physicians agree with this approach. Some "question the justification for the wide case-finding effort of subjecting asymptomatic persons to coronary arteriography . . . unless unusual findings suggest an especially poor prognosis" [3]. Others share this reluctance for an aggressive workup [4], while some take a middle of the road position that appears to leave open the possibility of coronary arteriographic study in appropriate patients with abnormal noninvasive tests [5].

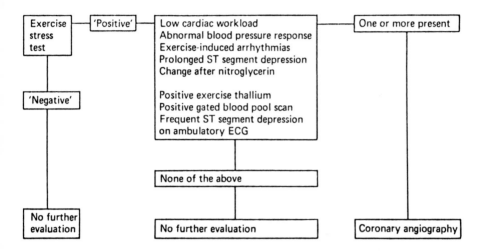

Figure 1 Flow diagram to illustrate one approach to evaluation of asymptomatic patients with a positive stress test. (From C. R. Conti. *Adv. Cardiol., 27*:181, 1980.)

II. INDICATIONS FOR CARDIAC CATHETERIZATION AFTER A MYOCARDIAL INFARCTION

Epstein et al. [6] have proposed a schema to identify patients who should undergo cardiac catheterization after a myocardial infarction (Figure 2). In addition to patients who are symptomatic with angina or congestive heart failure, they also recommend coronary arteriography in uncomplicated patients with adequate left ventricular function and inducible ischemia, i.e., ST segment depression and/or a fall in radionuclide ejection fraction. This recommendation is based on the adverse short-term prognosis associated with these findings. Veenbrink et al. [7] also used the exercise test response as a guide in their asymptomatic patients.

Mautner and Phillips [8] have a similar approach. They studied 31 patients, none (29%) of whom were found to have triple-vessel disease (Table 1). Chaitman et al. [9] found triple-vessel disease in 8 of 37 patients (22%), while Miller et al. (10] found this degree of obstruction in 38 of 84 patients (45%). Turner et al. [11] studied 117 patients with angiography—61 of whom were asymptomatic, i.e., uncomplicated—and found triple-vessel disease in 14 (29%), but also found left main disease in four (7%) (Table 2). Despite this high frequency of severe disease (36%), Turner et al. did *not* recommend routine coronary arteriography after a myocardial infarction

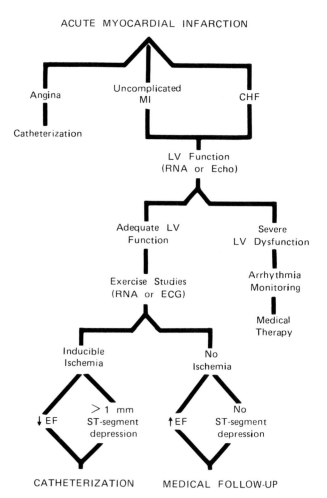

Figure 2 Strategy for identifying patients who should undergo cardiac catheter-ization after acute myocardial infarction. The strategy is based on clinical assess-ment, evaluation of left ventricular (LV) function by radionuclide angiography (RNA) or echocardiography, arrhythmia analysis, and stress testing. MI denotes acute myocardial infarction, CHF overt congestive heart failure and EF ejection fraction. (From S. E. Epstein, S. T. Palmeri, and R. E. Patterson. *N. Engl. J. Med.*, *307*:1487, 1982.)

Table 1 Coronary Arteriographic Findings

Left main disease	0
Left main equivalent	2 (6%)
Left anterior descending stenosis	22 (71%)
Inferior MI[a]	11
Anterior MI	11
Three vessel disease	9 (29%)
Two vessel disease	10 (32%)
Single vessel disease	10 (32%)
Normal	2 (6%)
Coronary artery aneurysms	1
Anomalous circumflex from right coronary artery	1
Absent collateral vessels	10 (32%)

[a]One proximal and nine distal to the first septal perforator.
Source: R. K. Mautner and J. H. Phillips. *Cardiovasc. Diag.*, 7:1, 1981.

because of the "uncertainty of bypass surgery in prolonging life" in this subgroup of patients.

III. INDICATIONS FOR CARDIAC CATHETERIZATION IN PATIENTS WITH BOTH SYMPTOMATIC AND ASYMPTOMATIC EPISODES OF MYOCARDIAL ISCHEMIA

The prevalence of this type of mixed picture varies from series to series but probably includes most anginal patients. In these patients, the factors that normally determine the decision to perform or not to perform coronary arteriography—refractoriness of symptoms, degree of abnormality of noninvasive tests—continue to be of prime importance. It is my belief, however, that we are rapidly reaching the point where consideration of the *total* number of ischemic episodes (symptomatic and silent) as documented by Holter monitoring will also be a determining factor in recommending both coronary arteriography and more aggressive management.

IV. CORONARY ARTERY DISEASE WITH AND WITHOUT SYMPTOMS: ARE THERE DISTINCTIVE ARTERIOGRAPHIC FEATURES?

One of the more intriguing questions concerning the pathophysiology of silent myocardial ischemia is whether there are any distinctive arteriographic

Table 2 Distribution of Coronary Artery Disease in Clinical Subsets of Postinfarction Patients

Distribution of coronary artery disease	Timing of angiography			Clinical convalescence		Infarction site			Extent of infarction	
	Early	Late	Total	Complicated	Uncomplicated	Anterior	Inferior	Indeterminate	Nontransmural	Transmural
Left main	10 (11)	0 (0)	10 (8.5)	6 (11)	4 (7)	3 (5)	7 (14)	0 (0)	1 (4)	9 (10)
3 vessels	28 (30)	13 (52)	41 (35)	22 (39)	19 (31)	27 (41)	14 (29)	0 (0)	10 (44)	31 (33)
2 vessels	29 (32)	8 (32)	37 (31.5)	15 (27)	22 (36)	17 (26)	18 (37)	2 (67)	6 (26)	31 (33)
1 vessel	23 (25)	4 (16)	27 (23)	12 (22)	15 (25)	17 (26)	9 (18)	1 (33)	5 (22)	22 (23)
0 vessels	2 (2)	0 (0)	2 (2)	1 (1)	1 (1)	1 (2)	1 (2)	0 (0)	1 (4)	1 (1)
Total	92 (100)	25 (100)	117 (100)	56 (100)	61 (100)	65 (100)	49 (100)	3 (100)	23 (100)	94 (100)

Percentages are shown in parentheses.
Source: J. D. Turner, W. J. Rogers, J. A. Mantel, C. E. Rackley, and R. O. Russell, Jr. *Chest*, 77:58, 1980.

features that help to identify patients with this phenomenon, or with silent myocardial infarction. Accordingly, pertinent data acquired in a number of studies will be reviewed.

Comparisons between *totally asymptomatic* Air Force personnel and angiographically normal persons are provided by Uhl and Froelicher [12]. The distribution of vessel disease in these patients is usually similar to that found in the symptomatic population. For example, Uhl reported that of the 65 men in his study, 32 had one-vessel disease, 17 had two-vessel disease, and 16 had three-vessel disease.

What of patients who are *asymptomatic following a myocardial infarction*? The study from the Duke-Harvard Collaborative Coronary Artery Disease Data Bank [13] can be used as a model for this kind of study since most of the patients had experienced a myocardial infarction. The clinical and angiographic findings in the 171 study patients (127 with and 44 without angina) were comparable. As we noted earlier in this chapter, Turner et al. [11], in a study of 92 asymptomatic postmyocardial infarction patients, found a 35% frequency of triple-vessel disease, 31.5% two-vessel disease, and 23% one-vessel disease. Mautner and Phillips [8] found a similar distribution (Table 1). When silent ischemia is clearly diagnosed on the basis of exercise testing, such as in the CASS registry, Weiner et al. [14] have shown no significant differences in prevalence of multivessel disease.

The final group to consider is patients with episodes of *both symptomatic and asymptomatic myocardial ischemia*. In one of the earliest studies, Lindsey and I [15] found multivessel disease in 75% of our patients. This compared to 83% (pNS) in patients who were symptomatic during a positive test. The prevalence of collateralization and low ejection fractions was also similar (Figure 3). Samek et al. [16] studied 102 patients with anginal histories but without angina on positive exercise test. Thirty-five percent had one-vessel disease, 32% two-vessel disease and 43% three-vessel disease. Most recently, Ouyang et al. [17] performed an angiographic comparison early after myocardial infarction in 60 consecutive patients with positive exercise tests (38, or 63%, had no pain and 22 had pain). No differences were found (Table 3). This is also the conclusion of a similar study by Falcone et al. [18].

Finally, let us consider patients with *silent myocardial infarctions*. Compared to patients with recognized myocardial infarctions, patients with clinically unrecognized myocardial infarctions have a similar extent of coronary artery disease, as determined by Gohlke et al. [19]. This is the same conclusion that Cabin and Roberts [20] reached in their autopsy study, which was discussed at greater length in Chapter 6.

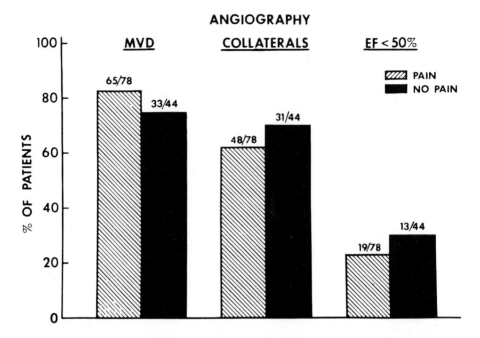

Figure 3 Frequency of multivessel disease (MVD), collateral vessels, and poor ventricular function in patients with and without angina pain. EF = ejection fraction. (From H. E. Lindsey, Jr., and P. F. Cohn. *Am. Heart J., 94*:441, 1978.)

In conclusion, it appears that there are no striking arteriographic differences between coronary artery disease patients with and without angina.

V. CORONARY ARTERIOGRAPHIC ASSESSMENT OF DIABETICS BEING EVALUATED FOR RENAL TRANSPLANTATION

Because athersclerotic cardiovascular disease is the most common cause of death in diabetic patients with severe renal disease, it has become accepted policy in many hospitals to clarify surgical risk by "screening" diabetic patients with noninvasive tests and/or cardiac catheterization. The findings are often quite dramatic. For example, Bennett et al. found severe coronary artery disease in all such patients in their study [21], while Weinrauch et al. [22] found severe coronary artery disease in 9 of 21 patients.

Table 3 Angiographic Characteristics in 60 Patients with Positive Early Post-infarction Exercise Tests[a]

	Silent treadmill ischemia (*n* = 38)	Symptomatic treadmill ischemia (*n* = 22)
	n (%)	*n* (%)
Left main disease	4 (11)	1 (6)
No. of CAs with ≥70% stenosis		
0	1 (3.6)	0 (0)
1	9 (24)	6 (27)
2	17 (45)	6 (27)
3	11 (29)	10 (45)
Totally occluded infarct artery	25 (66)	12 (55)
Coronary thrombus	28 (74)	12 (55)

[a]There is no significant difference between the two groups for any characteristic listed.
CAs = coronary arteries.
Source: P. Ouyang, E. P. Shapiro, N. C. Chandra, S. H. Gottlieb, P. H. Chew, and S. O. Gottlieb. *Am. J. Cardiol., 59*:730, 1987.

VI. CONCLUSIONS

Aside from treatment of asymptomatic persons, there is probably no more controversial area than indications for cardiac catheterization in totally asymptomatic individuals. Patients with positive exercise tests—generally those with early onset of ST changes and hypotension, or those who also have abnormal radionuclide studies—deserve aggressive follow-up with cardiac catheterization. Asymptomatic postinfarction patients with similar findings merit an equally aggressive approach, but this is less of an issue. Results of cardiac catheterization studies do not seem to indicate any particular angiographic patterns in any of the three types of silent ischemia patients when compared to symptomatic persons.

REFERENCES

1. J. A. Ambrose. Unsettled indications for coronary angiography. *J. Am. Coll. Cardiol., 3*:1575 (1984).
2. C. R. Conti. Detection and management of the asymptomatic patient with coronary artery disease. *Adv. Cardiol., 27*:181 (1980).

3. A. Selzer and K. Cohn. Asymptomatic coronary artery disease and coronary bypass surgery. *Am. J. Cardiol., 39*:614 (1977).

4. A. Rozanski and D. S. Berman. Silent myocardial ischemia: II. Prognosis and implications for the clinical assessment of patients with coronary artery disease. *Am. Heart J., 114*:627 (1987).

5. S. E. Epstein, A. A. Quyyumi, and R. O. Bonow. Myocardial ischemia— Silent or symptomatic. *N. Engl. J. Med., 318*:1039 (1988).

6. S. E. Epstein, S. T. Palmeri, and R. E. Patterson. Evaluation of patients after acute myocardial infarction. *N. Engl. J. Med., 307*:1487 (1982).

7. Th. W. G. Veenbrink, T. Van Der Werf, P. W. Westerhof, E. O. Robles deMedina, and F. L. Meijler. Is there an indication for coronary angiography in patients under 60 years of age with no or minimal angina pectoris after a first myocardial infarction? *Br. Heart J., 53*:30 (1985).

8. R. K. Mautner and J. H. Phillips. Coronary angiography post first myocardial infarction in the asymptomatic or mildly symptomatic patient: Clinical, angiographic, and prospective observations. *Cath. Cardiovasc. Diag., 7*:1 (1981).

9. B. R. Chaitman, D. Waters, F. Corbara, and M. Bourassa. Predictors of multivessel disease after inferior myocardial infarction. *Circulation, 57*:1085 (1978).

10. R. Miller, A. N. DeMaria, L. A. Vismara, et al.: Chronic stable inferior myocardial infarction: Unsuspected harbinger of high risk proximal left coronary arterial obstruction amenable to surgical revascularization. *Am. J. Cardiol., 39*:953 (1977).

11. J. D. Turner, W. J. Rogers, J. A. Mantle, C. E. Rackley, and R. O. Russell, Jr. Coronary angiography soon after myocardial infarction. *Chest, 77*:58 (1980).

12. G. S. Uhl and V. Froelicher. Screening for asymptomatic coronary artery disease. *J. Am. Coll. Cardiol., 1*:946 (1983).

13. P. F. Cohn, P. Harris, W. H. Barry, R. A. Rosati, P. Rosenbaum, and C. Waternaux. Prognostic importance of anginal symptoms in angiographically defined coronary artery disease. *Am. J. Cardiol., 47*:233 (1981).

14. D. A. Weiner, T. J. Ryan, C. H. McCabe, S. Luk, B. R. Chaitman, L. T. Sheffield, F. Tristani, and L. D. Fisher. Significance of silent myocardial ischemia during exercise testing in patients with coronary artery disease. *Am. J. Cardiol., 49*:725 (1987).

15. H. E. Lindsey, Jr., and P. F. Cohn. "Silent" myocardial ischemia during and after exercise testing in patients with coronary artery disease. *Am. Heart J., 94*:441 (1978).

16. L. Samek, P. Beta, and H. Roskamm. ST-segment depression during exercise without angina pectoris in postinfarction patients: Angiographic findings and prognostic relevance. In *Silent Myocardial Ischemia* (W. Rutishauser and H. Roskamm, eds.), Springer-Verlag, Berlin, 1984, pp. 170-175.

17. P. Ouyang, E. P. Shapiro, N. C. Chandra, S. H. Gottlieb, P. H. Chew, and S. O. Gottlieb. An angiographic and functional comparison of patients with silent and symptomatic treadmill ischemia early after myocardial infarction. *Am. J. Cardiol., 59*:730 (1987).

18. C. Falcone, S. DeServi, E. Pom, C. Campana, A. Scire, C. Montemartini, and G. Specchia. Clinical significance of exercise-induced silent myocardial ischemia in patients with coronary artery disease. *J. Am. Coll. Cardiol., 9*: 295 (1987).

19. H. Gohlke, K. Peters, P. Betz, P. Sturzenhofecker, E. Steinmann, T. Vellguth, and H. Roskamm. Angiography in patients with silent myocardial infarction. In *Silent Myocardial Ischemia* (W. Rutishauser and H. Roskamm, eds.), Springer-Verlag, Berlin, 1984, pp. 138-143.

20. H. S. Cabin and W. C. Roberts. Quantitative comparison of extent of coronary narrowing and size of healed myocardial infarct in 33 necropsy patients with clinically unrecognized ("silent") previous acute myocardial infarction. *Am. J. Cardiol., 50*:677 (1982).

21. W. M. Bennett, F. Kloster, J. Rosch, J. Barry, and G. A. Porter. Natural history of asymptomatic coronary arteriographic lesions in diabetic patients with end-stage renal disease. *Am. J. Med., 65*:779 (1978).

22. T. Weinrauch, J. A. D'Elia, R. W. Healy, R. E. Gleason, A. R. Christlieb, and O. S. Leland, Jr. Asymptomatic coronary artery disease: Angiographic assessment of diabetics evaluated for renal transplantation. *Circulation, 58*: 1184 (1978).

IV
PROGNOSIS IN ASYMPTOMATIC CORONARY ARTERY DISEASE

12

Prognosis in Patients with Silent Myocardial Ischemia

Silent myocardial ischemia is a ubiquitous phenomenon; therefore, any discussion of prognosis quickly becomes mired down in confusion if groups of patients are not clearly differentiated. As noted earlier in this book, since 1981 we consider this phenomenon in three types of patients. One group consists of individuals who have never had symptoms (Type 1), the second group consists of individuals who are asymptomatic following a myocardial infarction but still manifest ischemia (Type 2) and the third group includes individuals who are symptomatic with some of their ischemic episodes but not with others (Type 3). The latter can be further divided into patients with chronic versus unstable angina pectoris.

I. PROGNOSIS IN TOTALLY ASYMPTOMATIC INDIVIDUALS

Data in individuals of this type who also have angiographically confirmed disease is especially hard to come by, since physicians are naturally reluctant to submit asymptomatic individuals to a potentially dangerous invasive procedure. One of the few surveys that have provided a large series of subjects is that conducted by the U.S. Air Force School of Aerospace Medicine in San Antonio, Texas. The Air Force survey, commented on earlier in this book, was begun by Froelicher and colleagues in the mid-1970s [1]. Cardiac catheterization was performed on asymptomatic airmen with abnormal treadmill tests, as described in Chapters 9 and 10. Subsequent treadmill or radionuclide studies, or both, performed by Uhl and Froelicher [2] and later by Uhl et al. [3] resulted in a total of 78 asymptomatic airmen with significant coronary artery disease being detected. Along with 12 other airmen with minimal coronary artery disease, this group was followed for several years to evaluate those factors influencing prognosis.

In their 1980 report from the San Antonio survey, Hickman et al. [4] noted that 22 of the 78 airmen with significant disease (more than 50% luminal stenosis) developed overt signs of coronary artery disease, i.e., angina, myocardial infarction, death within a 4-90-month follow-up period. The mean time was 57 months and the men ranged in age from 47 to 54 years. Of the 22 with significant coronary artery disease, 16 developed angina at a mean duration of 31.5 months, four sustained a myocardial infarction and two died suddenly. In addition to the 22, six other men developed symptoms at a later time (mean age 46 months). Of these six, five developed angina and one died suddenly. The authors investigated the influence of the four standard coronary risk factors (cigarette smoking, hyperlipidemia, diabetes and hypertension) and found that at least three of these risk factors were present in nearly half of the men who had subsequent cardiac events. These provocative findings highlight the importance of risk factors in prognosis of asymptomatic men, as well as in the screening of such populations, as previously discussed in Part III.

In the smaller series reported by Langou et al. [5] from Yale University, the authors followed their 12 subjects with significant coronary artery

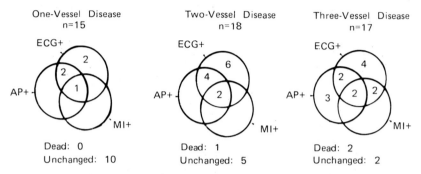

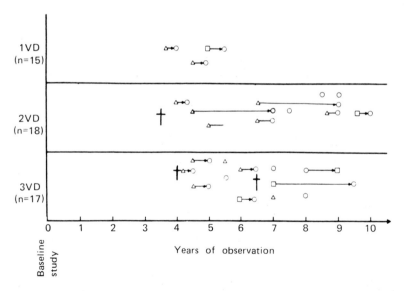

Figure 1 Venn diagrams showing the relation between baseline angiographic findings and coronary artery disease (CAD) events during a mean follow-up of 8½ years in 50 men with asymptomatic CAD. AP = angina pectoris. (From J. Erikssen and E. Thaulow. In *Silent Myocardial Ischemia* [W. Rutishauser and H. Roskamm, eds.], Springer-Verlag, Berlin, 1984, pp. 156-164.)

Figure 2 CAD progression in relation to baseline coronary angiographic findings and years of follow-up in 50 men with asymptomatic CAD diagnosed at the baseline study. Arrow length indicates the interval between first CAD event and coronary angiographic verification of CAD progression. † = death; O = angiographic progression; □ = myocardial infarction; Δ = AP. (From J. Erikssen and E. Thaulow. In *Silent Myocardial Ischemia* [W. Rutishauser and H. Roskamm, eds.], Springer-Verlag, Berlin, 1984, pp. 156-164.)

disease for three years. In that period of time, three men developed angina and one a myocardial infarction, though none died.

The most ambitious of all of these studies ws the one performed in Norway by Erikssen and colleagues [6,7]. From a large cohort of men aged 40-50 years who underwent a comprehensive cardiovascular screening in 1972-1975, 60 were identified as having significant coronary artery disease, 18 with one-vessel disease, 25 with two-vessel disease and 26 with three-vessel disease. Fifty of the sixty-nine men were unequivocally felt to have asymptomatic coronary artery disease; in the other 19, it was questionable whether mild symptoms were present. After an eight-to-ten-year period of following the 50 asymptomatic men, the authors found that three died from cardiac disease and seven had a myocardial infarction (five of which were silent). In addition, as depicted in Figure 1, 16 other men developed angina pectoris. Twenty-four patients had repeat angiograms; 23 of the 24 had progression (56%) (Figure 2) and 11 underwent coronary bypass surgery. Thus, a total of 28 (56%) of the 50 men either died, had a myocardial infarction, developed angina or had progression on coronary angiography. (Men with and without these events were of similar age, had similar heart rates and blood pressure.) The total mortality was less than 1%/year, but this may be skewered by the 11 men sent for bypass surgery. Clinical events were observed mostly in men with multivessel disease. The authors concluded that once they are diagnosed, subjects with asymptomatic coronary artery disease should be followed yearly. In that manner, rapid detection of clinical events is possible and appropriate thereapy can be initiated. This is usually conservative, though the authors infer that patients with left main disease—like their symptomatic counterparts—should be offered aggressive management in light of the "malignant" course of the five patients in the study—two dead and three others with angiographic or clinical progression. The importance of close follow-up is emphasized by the most recent report from the Norwegian survey [8]. At the 12-year mark, there were now four deaths in the two-vessel disease group and six in the three-vessel disease subgroup. Thus, the yearly mortality in the latter patients approaches 3%.

Another interesting subgroup of asymptomatic patients are those with diabetes mellitus and end-stage renal disease who are being considered for transplantation. Bennett et al. [9] reported on 11 consecutive patients (previously discussed in Chapter 11), eight of whom died within the 20-month mean follow-up period; six died of cardiac causes (Table 1).

In the nonangiographic group, several epidemiologic studies have called attention to the increased mortality associated with positive exercise tests in asymptomatic persons (see Chapter 9).

Table 1 Clinical Course of Asymptomatic Diabetic Patients with Coronary Arteriographic Abnormalities

Case no.	Duration of follow-up to death or to present analysis (mo)	Modality of renal disease treatment	Outcome of therapy	Pathology	Worsening of hyperlipo-proteinemia	Comments
1	30	Rejection of two cadaver transplants	Alive on dialysis	—	Yes	—
2	18	Cadaver transplant	Death from stroke	Diffuse coronary arterio-sclerosis	No	Normal renal function at time of death
3	7	Live donor transplant	Death from sepsis and cardiac arrest	No necropsy	No	Normal renal function at time of death
4	12	Long-term hemodialysis	Death while on machine	No necropsy	Yes	History of chest pain and drop in blood pressure prior to death
5	38	Long-term dialysis	Alive	—	No	Angina pectoris when hematocrit less than 25%
6	28	Long-term dialysis	Death from myocardial infarct	Extensive coronary disease, fresh infarct	No	Infarct 6 hours after dialysis treatment

Table 1 (Continues)

Table 1 Continued

Case no.	Duration of follow-up to death or to present analysis (mo)	Modality of renal disease treatment	Outcome of therapy	Pathology	Worsening of hyperlipoproteinemia	Comments
7	36	Related donor transplant	Alive	—	No	Angina pectoris for 6 mo. hypertension and decreased graft function due to graft arteriosclerosis
8	18	Long-term dialysis	Death from infarct and pulmonary edema	No necropsy	Yes	—
9	4	Long-term dialysis	Death from massive myocardial infarct	No necropsy	No	Major gastrointestinal hemorrhage preceded fatal event
10	11	Cadaver transplant	Death from myocardial infarct	Confirmed coronary disease postmortem	No	Rejection, uremic pericarditis preceded fatal event
11	16	Long-term dialysis	Death following coronary vein bypass surgery	Fresh myocardial infarct	Yes	Disabling angina; marked progression demonstrated on preoperative angiogram

Source: W. B. Bennett, F. Kloster, J. Rosch, J. Barry, and G. A. Porter. *Am. J. Med.*, 65:779, 1979.

II. PROGNOSIS IN PATIENTS WHO ARE ASYMPTOMATIC FOLLOWING A MYOCARDIAL INFARCTION

These studies usually have heterogeneous populations. For example, an investigation at the National Institutes of Health (NIH) followed 20 patients who were asymptomatic after an infarction but included five other totally asymptomatic persons and 122 mildly asymptomatic persons (61 of whom had prior infarctions) in their study group [10]. As expected, there was a high frequency of coronary risk factors in this group. Thus, 90 patients were (or had been) cigarette smokers, 33 had hypertension, 22 had hypercholesterolemia and 48 had either clinical diabetes or an abnormal glucose tolerance test. Forty-one of the patients had single-vessel coronary artery disease (28%), 45 had double-vessel disease (31%), and 61 had triple-vessel disease (41%). In the entire group, the authors could not find any combination of *clinical* risk factors that identified a high-risk subgroup, and the entire group mortality was 3%/year, a figure lower

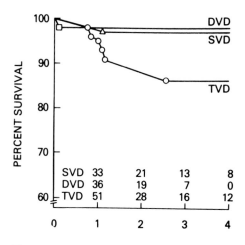

Figure 3 Life-table analysis of 147 patients with single- (SVD), double- (DVD) and triple-vessel (TVD) coronary artery disease for up to 4 years after entry into the study. Eight deaths occurred during the follow-up period at which time the probability data were generated. The line is extended to 4 years in each group after the last death occurred, although this is an extrapolation and not based on another set of probability data. The number of patients in the study at each yearly interval in each subgroup are shown at botton. (From K. M. Kent, D. R. Rosing, C. J. Ewels, L. Lipson, R. Bonow, and S. E. Epstein. *Am. J. Cardiol., 49*:1823, 1982.)

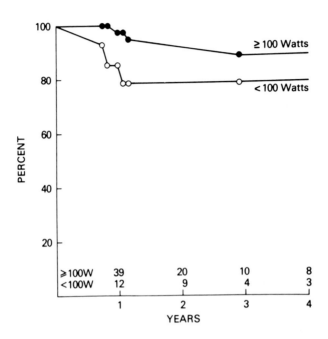

Figure 4 Life-table analysis comparing patients with triple-vessel disease who were able to achieve 100 or more watts on the bicycle ergometer and patients who had poor exercise capacity (less than 100 watts). In this comparison between two groups, probability data are calculated for both groups when an event occurs in either group. (From K. M. Kent, D. R. Rosing, C. J. Ewels, L. Lipson, R. Bonow, and S. E. Epstein. *Am. J. Cardiol., 49*:1823, 1982.)

than reported for symptomatic groups. The life-table analysis of the entire cohort of 147 patients is depicted in Figure 3. In the four years of follow-up, eight deaths occurred. The triple-vessel group was studied separately. Figure 4 shows that patients with good exercise capacity had an annual mortality of 4%, while those with poor exercise capacity had an annual mortality of 9%; total mortality was 6%. (This compared to 3% in the Norwegian survey of asymptomatic patients without prior infarctions [8].) In a follow-up study at the NIH, the authors evaluated only patients with resting ejection fractions >0.40 (new patients with ejection fractions >0.40 were also added). The purpose of the new study of 117 patients was "to test the hypothesis that in patients with preserved left ventricular function at rest, the presence and severity of reversible ischemia (measured by both radionuclide angiography and exercise electrocardiography) may be a more specific predictor of prognosis during medical therapy." The authors found that patients with three-vessel disease, positive ST segment response to exercise, exercise capacity less than 120 watts and an exercise-induced fall in ejection fraction had an annual mortality rate of 7% [11], confirming their hypotheses. In their most recent series of 131 patients with ejection fractions >0.40 (53 of whom had prior infarctions) they concentrated on patients with left main and triple-vessel disease [12]. They found that in patients with both a decrease in radionuclide ejection fraction during exercise and ST depression, there was a similar percentage of left main and triple vessel disease in both the angina and non-angina groups (Figure 5); the death rate in these patients was also similar. The authors concluded that "Once inducible ischemia is demonstrated, the symptomatic response to exercise, by itself, appears irrelevant for risk stratification considerations." These conclusions are confirmed by the experience from the Coronary Artery Surgery Study (CASS) registry, which consists largely of asymptomatic or mildly symptomatic post-

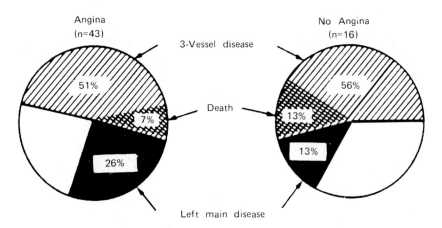

Figure 5 Prevalence of left main and three-vessel disease among patients with both a decrease in ejection fraction (EF) and a positive ST-segment response. Patients are subdivided on the basis of symptomatic vs silent ischemia during exercise. Patients with these ischemic responses had a similar likelihood of three-vessel disease, left main disease, and death during medical therapy, regardless of the presence or absence of angina during exercise. (From R. O. Bonow, S. L. Bacharach, M. V. Green, R. L. LaFreniere, and S. E. Epstein. *Am. J. Cardiol., 60*:778, 1987.)

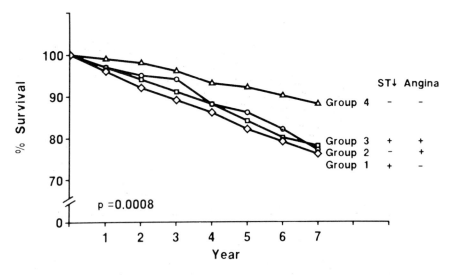

Figure 6   Cumulative survival for patients in groups 1 through 4. The 7-year survival was similar to patients in groups 1 (the silent ischemia group), 2, and 3. Group 4 patients (with neither angina nor ST depression) had a substantially better 7-year survival. (From D. A. Weiner, T. J. Ryan, C. H. McCabe, S. Luk, B. R. Chaitman, L. T. Sheffield, F. Tristani, and L. D. Fisher. *Am. J. Cardiol., 59*: 725, 1987.)

infarction patients. In a 1987 report, Weiner et al. [13] found painless exercise-induced ischemia to carry the same prognosis as painful ischemia (Figure 6). When the severity of coronary artery disease is considered, the group with three-vessel disease had a 6% yearly mortality (Figure 7), similar to the prior figures from the NIH group.

Another study that arrived at a similar percentage was reported several years earlier by the Duke-Harvard Collaborative Coronary Artery Disease Data Bank [14]. This survey also included a mixture of totally asymptomatic and partially asymptomatic patients with angiographically documented coronary artery disease. Thirty-two had prior infarctions. The 44 patients were matched with 127 symptomatic patients from the same data bank. The computerized matching process was based on five variables that reflected coronary anatomy and left ventricular function. Originally we had hoped to match each of the 44 asymptomatic patients with three symptomatic patients to ensure a large enough data base, but this was not always possible; hence, the final figure for the control group was 127

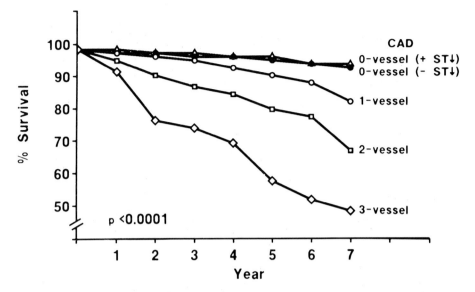

Figure 7 Seven-year survival rates for group 1 patients in Figure 6 based on the severity of coronary artery disease (CAD); a separate group of 282 patients without CAD who had ischemic ST-segment depression (+ ST↓) without angina during exercise testing; and a control group of 1,117 patients without CAD and without either ischemic ST depression (– ST↓) or angina during exercise testing. (From D. A. Weiner, T. J. Ryan, C. H. McCabe, S. Luk, B. R. Chaitman, L. T. Sheffield, F. Tristani, and L. D. Fisher. *Am. J. Cardiol., 59*:725, 1987.)

rather than 132. In addition to the five variables noted earlier, we also compared the frequency of other variables once the groups were selected by the computer. This was to insure that the results of the survival analysis were not influenced by descriptors that were not selected to be matched by the computer. This comparison is depicted in Table 2; there were no significant differences between the two groups. Mean follow-up time was 3 1/2 years. There was an 81% survival rate for the total asymptomatic group at seven years (yearly mortality 2.7%), compared with a 62% survival rate for the symptomatic group (yearly mortality 5.4%). The worst prognosis was in the subgroup with three-vessel disease (4.7% vs. 8.7% in the symptomatic group) (Figure 8). Two of the four patients in the symptomatic group who died had anginal symptoms at least six months before their death; development of anginal symptoms eventually was reported in 30% of the patients by the end of the 4-year follow-up.

Table 2 Clinical and Angiographic Findings in Study Patients With and Without Anginal Symptoms

	Without anginal symptoms ($n = 44$)	With anginal symptoms ($n = 127$)
Mean age	47.6	49.0
Male sex	41 (93%)	107 (84%)
Diabetes	2 (4%)	8 (6%)
Hypertension	13 (29%)	27 (21%)
Diagnostic Q waves in electrocardiogram	23 (53%)	76 (60%)
Positive exercise test	17/31 (55%)	48/96 (50%)
Two vessel disease	13 (30%)	38 (30%)
Three vessel disease	18 (40%)	51 (40%)
Left main coronary arterial stenosis	0	0
Left anterior descending arterial stenosis	36 (82%)	91 (72%)
Totally occluded vessels	12 (27%)	34 (27%)
Abnormal left ventricular contraction pattern	32 (73%)	95 (75%)
Left ventricular end-diastolic pressure > 18 mmHg	8 (18%)	18 (14%)
Arteriovenous oxygen difference > 5.5 volumes percent	9 (21%)	23 (18%)

Source: P. F. Cohn, P. Harris, W. H. Barry, R. A. Rosati, P. Rosenbaum, and C. Waternaux. *Am. J. Cardiol.*, 47:233, 1981.

In addition to these studies, there are numerous reports describing prognosis in patients who have sustained an *acute* myocardial infarction. Short-term survival statistics based on the post-infarction exercise studies indicate that exercise-induced ST segment depression markedly increases the 1-year mortality. In some of these studies, prognosis in those patients who were asymptomatic and had positive exercise tests denoting active, though silent, myocardial ischemia could be gleaned from the raw data. For example, in the study by Theroux et al. [15], 210 patients who had no overt heart failure and had been free of chest pain for at least 4 days were exercised one day before discharge from the hospital. The 1-year mortality rate was 2.1% (3 of 146) in patients without ischemic ST changes during exercise and 27% (17 of 64) in those with such changes ($p < 0.001$). The authors reported that angina in the presence of ST segment depression had no effect on these statistics. Thus, 10 of 37 patients with ST depression on the exercise test but without angina died, compared with 7 of 27

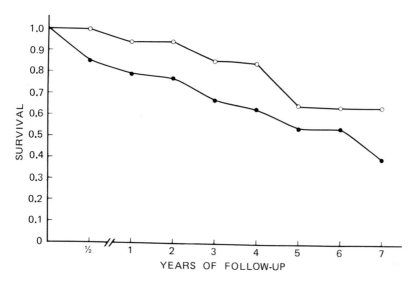

Figure 8 Survival curves for 17 patients (O) with three-vessel coronary artery disease but without angina symptoms compared to 49 patients (●) with three-vessel disease and anginal symptoms, in the Duke-Harvard Coronary Artery Disease (CAD) Data Bank.

with both exercise-induced ST depression and angina. More recently, Gibson and Beller [16] have reported that postinfarction patients with painless exercise ST depression at the highest risk for future cardiac events are those with thallium-201 redistribution defects.

Holter data in the postinfarction patient is still limited, but several recent studies indicate that the presence of silent ischemia on Holter monitoring can predict mortality [17,18].

Other prognostic studies involving therapy are discussed subsequently in Section V.

III. PROGNOSIS IN PATIENTS WITH BOTH SYMPTOMATIC AND ASYMPTOMATIC ISCHEMIC EPISODES

Several studies have investigated the prognosis of patients with *chronic angina* who have a positive exercise test without pain. (Usually a painful but positive test remains so with repeat testing some months later [19]). Presumably, these individuals have both symptomatic and silent ischemic episodes during daily activities. Rabaeus et al. [20] studied 150 such patients with coronary artery disease, 40 with prior infarction but no cardiac catheterization and 110 who were catheterized. Forty-three patients had one-vessel disease, 37 had two-vessel disease, and 30 had three-vessel disease. Mean follow-up time was 45 months. Major coronary events (unstable angina, myocardial infarction, coronary artery bypass surgery or sudden death) occurred in 76 patients (51%). These events were significantly associated with extent of coronary artery disease. When correlations with other factors during the exercise test were made between these 76 patients and the 74 without major coronary events, no positive relationship was noted.

Samek et al. [21] studied 102 patients post infarction (23 with one-vessel disease, 31 with two-vessel disease, and 48 with three-vessel disease). The 5-year mortality rate in 72 medically treated patients was 7% and the rate of cardiac events (death or nonfatal myocardial infarction) was 12%. Samek et al. compared these figures to those of a larger group of 325 patients with both ischemic changes and angina during testing. Mortality in this symptomatic control group was 16% and the rate of cardiac events 21%. The authors concluded that prognosis was better in patients *without* angina during positive exercise tests. Rabeus, et al. had no such control group. Three other recent studies have also examined prognosis in patients with chronic angina. Falcone et al. [22] compared follow-up in 269 patients with painful ischemia during exercise to 204 patients with painless ischemia. Several curves were similar regardless of the symptoms (Figure 9). Dagenais et al. [23] reported similar findings in 298 patients with strongly positive exercise tests. By contrast, Assey et al. [24] found a worse prognosis in their series of 55 patients studied with exercise thallium scintography (Table 3) when pain was absent. Not all prognostic studies need rely on exercise testing. The first reports are now available concerning follow-up results in patients subjected to long-term ambulatory monitoring (as described in Chapter 8). These reports show that Holter evidence of ischemia adds important incremental data to that obtained from the clinical history and/or a positive exercise test [25,26].

Figure 9 Survival curves of medically treated patients with (Group I) (*dashed lines*) or without (Group II) (*solid lines*) angina during stress testing. No statistically significant difference was found between the two groups even when patients were classified according to the number of disease. (From C. Falcone, S. DeServi, E. Poma, C. Campana, A. Scire, C. Montemartini, and G. Specchia. *J. Am. Coll. Cardiol.*, 9:295, 1987.)

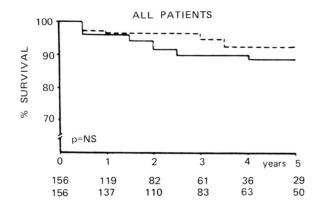

ALL PATIENTS

0	1	2	3	4	5
156	119	82	61	36	29
156	137	110	83	63	50

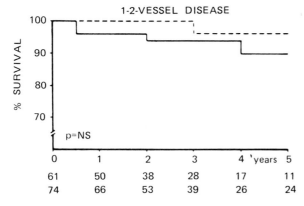

1-2-VESSEL DISEASE

0	1	2	3	4	5
61	50	38	28	17	11
74	66	53	39	26	24

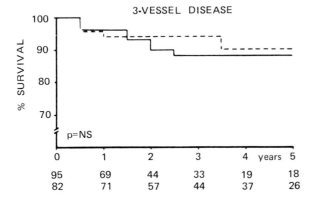

3-VESSEL DISEASE

0	1	2	3	4	5
95	69	44	33	19	18
82	71	57	44	37	26

Table 3 Cardiac Events of Study Population During Follow-Up

Event	Group I (n = 27)	Group II (n = 28)	p value
Acute MI	6 (22%)	1 (4%)	0.05
Death	3 (11%)	0 (0%)	NS
Hospitalization for unstable angina	13 (48%)	16 (57%)	NS

MI = myocardial infarction; NS = not significantly different.
Source: M. E. Assey, G. L. Waters, G. H. Hendrix, B. A. Carabello, B. W. Usher, and J. F. Spann, Jr. *Am. J. Cardiol., 59*:497, 1987.

Table 4 Two-Year Adverse Clinical Outcomes for Unstable Angina Patients With and Without Silent ST Segment Changes on Initial 48 Hour Holter Monitoring

Adverse clinical outcome	Group I: Silent ischemia (n = 37)		Group II: No silent ischemia (n = 33)		p value[a]
Cardiac death	2	(27%)	0	(3%)	<0.01
Nonfatal MI	8		1		
CABG or PTCA for symptoms	11	(30%)	5	(15%)	<0.05
Total	21	(57%)	6	(18%)	<0.001

[a]Derived from Kaplan-Meier analysis, Breslow test.
CAGB = coronary bypass surgery; MI = myocardial infarction; PTCA = percutaneous transluminal coronary angioplasty.
Source: S. O. Gottlieb, M. L. Weisfeldt, P. Ouyang, E. D. Mellits, and G. Gerstenblith. *J. Am. Coll. Cardiol., 10*:756, 1987.

Additional Holter data is also available in patients with unstable angina. Gottlieb et al. studied 70 patients with this syndrome; 37 had Holter ECG evidence of silent ischemia, 33 did not. Thirty-day [27] and two-year [28] follow-up showed a significant pattern of adverse events associated with silent ischemia (Table 4) but not with negative Holter findings (Figure 10). Similar findings were reported by Nademanee et al. [29], who also confirmed the importance of more than 60 min of ischemia/per 24 hr of Holter monitoring (Figure 11).

IV. CONCLUSIONS

In general, prognosis in totally asymptomatic individuals with silent myocardial ischemia appears good, the exception being those with three-vessel

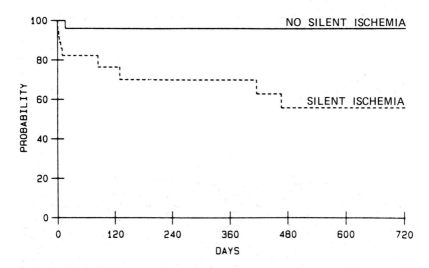

Figure 10 Kaplan-Meier curves illustrating the probabilities of *not* experiencing death or myocardial infarction over the 2 year follow-up period for the 37 patients with (Group I) and the 33 patients without (Group II) silent ischemic ST changes on initial Holter monitoring. The difference between the two groups is significant at the *p* < 0.01 level. (From S. O. Gottlieb, M. L. Weisfeldt, P. Ouyang, E. D. Mellits, and G. Gerstenblith. *J. Am. Coll. Cardiol., 10*:756, 1987.)

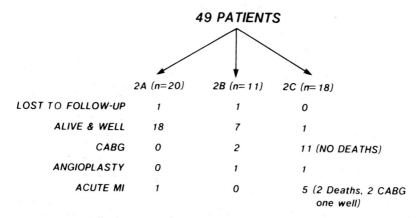

Figure 11 Flow diagram demonstrating the clinical outcome of 49 patients with unstable angina relative to the presence and duration of transient myocardial ischemia (TMI) in patients with unstable angina. CABG = coronary artery bypass surgery; MI = myocardial infarction. Patients were subgrouped as follows: 2A = no transient myocardial ischemia; 2B and 2C = transient myocardial ischemia < 60 min/24 hr and > 60 min/24 hr, respectively. (From K. Nadamanee, V. Intarachot, M. A. Josephson, D. Rieders, F. V. Mody, and B. N. Singh. *J. Am. Coll. Cardiol., 19*:1, 1987.)

181

disease. Similarly, patients who are asymptomatic after an infarction contain a subgroup of individuals with three-vessel disease who have far from a benign prognosis. Mortality in this group averages 6%. What effect the presence of frequent silent ischemic episodes has on the prognosis of patients with chronic angina is still unresolved, but exercise test data indicates prognosis is similar with exercise-induced ST depression whether angina is present or not. Holter data in unstable angina indicates that continuing ischemia, which is usually silent ischemia, has an adverse effect on cardiovascular morbidity and mortality.

REFERENCES

1. V. F. Froelicher, A. J. Thompson, M. R. Longo, J. Triebwasser, and M. C. Lancaster. Value of exercise testing for screening asymptomatic men for latent coronary heart disease. *Prog. Cardiovasc. Dis., 18*:265 (1976).

2. G. S. Uhl and V. Froelicher. Screening for asymptomatic coronary artery disease. *J. Am. Coll. Cardiol., 1*:946 (1983).

3. G. S. Uhl, T. N. Kay, and J. R. Hickman, Jr. Comparison of exercise radionuclide angiography and thallium perfusion imaging in detecting coronary disease in asymptomatic men. *J. Cardiac Rehabil., 2*:118 (1982).

4. J. R. Hickman, Jr., G. S. Uhl, R. L. Cook, P. J. Engel, and A. Hopkirk. A natural history study of asymptomatic coronary disease (abstr). *Am. J. Cardiol., 45*:422 (1980).

5. R. A. Langou, E. K. Huang, M. J. Kelley, and L. D. Cohen. Predictive accuracy of coronary artery calcification and abnormal exercise test for coronary artery disease in asymptomatic men. *Circulation, 62*:1196 (1980).

6. J. Erikssen and E. Thaulow. Follow-up of patients with asymptomatic myocardial ischemia. In *Silent Myocardial Ischemia* (W. Rutishauser and H. Roskamm, eds.), Springer-Verlag, Berlin, 1984, pp. 156-164.

7. J. Erikssen and R. Mundal. The patient with coronary disease without infarction: Can a high risk group be identified? *Ann. NY Acad. Sci., 382*:483 (1982).

8. J. Erikssen, E. Thaulow, and P. F. Cohn. Long-term prognosis of fifty totally asymptomatic middle-aged men with silent myocardial ischemia and angiographically documented coronary artery disease (abstr). *Circulation, 76*(Suppl IV):77 (1987).

9. W. M. Bennett, F. Kloster, J. Rosch, J. Barry, and G. A. Porter. Natural history of asymptomatic coronary arteriographic lesions in diabetic patients with end-stage renal disease. *Am. J. Med., 65*:779 (1978).

10. K. M. Kent, D. R. Rosing, C. J. Ewes, L. Lipson, R. Bonow, and S. E. Epstein. Prognosis of asymptomatic or mildly symptomatic patients with coronary artery disease. *Am. J. Cardiol., 49*:1823 (1982).

11. R. O. Bonow, K. M. Kent, D. R. Rosing, K. K. G. Lan, E. Lakatos, J. S. Borer, S. L. Bacharach, M. V. Green, and S. E. Epstein. Exercise-induced ischemia in mildly symptomatic patients with coronary artery disease and preserved left ventricular function: Identification of subgroups at risk of death during medical therapy. *N. Engl. J. Med., 311*:1339 (1984).

12. R. O. Bonow, S. L. Bacharach, M. V. Green, R. L. LaFreniere, and S. E. Epstein. Prognostic implications of symptomatic versus asymptomatic (silent) myocardial ischemia induced by exercise in mildly symptomatic and in asymptomatic patients with angiographically documented coronary artery disease. *Am. J. Cardiol., 60*:778 (1987).

13. D. A. Weiner, T. J. Ryan, C. H. McCabe, S. Luk, B. R. Chaitman, L. T. Sheffield, F. Tristani, and L. D. Fisher. Significance of silent myocardial ischemia during exercise testing in patients with coronary artery disease. *Am. J. Cardiol., 59*:725 (1987).

14. P. F. Cohn, P. Harris, W. H. Barry, R. Rosati, P. Rosenbaum, and C. Waternaux. Prognostic importance of anginal symptoms in angiographically defined coronary artery disease. *Am. J. Cardiol., 47*:233 (1981).

15. P. Theroux, D. D. Waters, C. Halphen, J. C. Debaisieux, and H. F. Mizgala. Prognostic value of exercise testing soon after myocardial infarction. *N. Engl. J. Med., 301*:341 (1979).

16. R. S. Gibson and G. A. Beller. Prevalence and clinical significance of painless ST segment depression during early post infarction exercise testing. *Circulation, 75*(Suppl II):II-36 (1987).

17. S. O. Gottlieb, S. H. Gottlieb, S. C. Achuff, R. Baumgardner, E. D. Mellits, M. L. Weisfeldt, and G. Gerstenblith. Silent ischemia on Holter monitoring predicts mortality in high-risk postinfarction patients. *J.A.M.A., 259*:1030 (1988).

18. D. Tzivoni, A. Gavish, D. Zin, S. Gottlieb, Mady Moriel, A. Keren, S. Banai, and S. Stern. Prognostic significance of ischemic episodes in patients with previous myocardial infarction. *Am. J. Cardiol., 62*:661 (1988).

19. G. Weisz, S. Stern, and D. Tzivoni. Is a silent or painful treadmill test predictive of a silent or painful treadmill test repeated one year later? *Circulation, 76*(Suppl IV):361 (1987).

20. M. Rabaeus, A. Righetti, and P. Moret. Long-term follow-up of patients with positive exercise test without angina in a referred population. In *Silent Myocardial Ischemia* (W. Rutishauser and H. Roskamm, eds.), Springer-Verlag, Berlin, 1984, pp. 165-169.

21. L. Samek, P. Betz, and H. Roskamm. ST-segment depression during exercise without angina pectoris in postinfarction patients: Angiographic findings and prognostic relevance. In *Silent Myocardial Ischemia* (W. Rutishauser and H. Roskamm, eds.), Springer-Verlag, Berlin, 1984, pp. 170-175.

22. C. Falcone, S. deServi, E. Poma, C. Campana, A. Scire, C. Montemartini, and G. Specchia. Clinical significance of exercise-induced silent myocardial

ischemia in patients with coronary artery disease. *J. Am. Coll. Cardiol., 9*: 295 (1987).

23. G. Dagenais, J. R. Rouleau, P. Hochart, J. Magrina, B. Cantin, and J. G. Dumesnil. Survival with painless strongly positive exercise electrocardiogram. *Am. J. Cardiol. 62*:892 (1988).

24. M. E. Assey, G. L. Walters, G. H. Hendrix, B. A. Crabello, B. W. Usher, and J. F. Spann, Jr. Incidence of acute myocardial infarction in patients with exercise-induced silent myocardial ischemia. *Am. J. Cardiol., 59*:497 (1987).

25. M. B. Rocco, E. G. Nabel, S. Campbell, L. Goldman, J. Barry, K. Mead, and A. P. Selwyn. Prognostic importance of myocardial ischemia detected by ambulatory monitoring in patients with coronary disease (abstr). *J. Am. Coll. Cardiol., 9*:68A (1987).

26. P. Deedwania, E. Carbajai, and J. Nelson. Silent ischemia during Holter monitoring: A marker of mortality and adverse clinical outcome in stable angina (abstr). *Circulation, 78*(Suppl II):II-43 (1988).

27. S. O. Gottlieb, M. L. Weisfeldt, P. Ouyang, E. D. Mellits, and G. Gerstenblith. Silent ischemia as a marker for early unfavorable outcomes in patients with unstable angina. *N. Engl. J. Med., 314*:1214 (1986).

28. S. O. Gottlieb, M. L. Weisfeldt, P. Ouyang, E. D. Mellits, and G. Gerstenblith. Silent ischemia predicts infarction and death during 2 year follow-up of unstable angina. *J. Am. Coll. Cardiol., 19*:756 (1987).

29. K. Nademanee, V. Intarachot, M. A. Josephson, D. Rieders, F. V. Mody, and B. N. Singh. Prognostic significance of silent myocardial ischemia in patients with unstable angina. *J. Am. Coll. Cardiol., 19*:1 (1987).

13

Relation of Silent Myocardial Ischemia to Sudden Death, Silent Myocardial Infarction, and Ischemic Cardiomyopathy

In addition to the overall prognostic picture provided in Chapter 12, there are three potential complications of silent myocardial ischemia that warrant special comment: sudden death, silent myocardial infarction and ischemic cardiomyopathy.

I. SILENT MYOCARDIAL ISCHEMIA, VENTRICULAR ARRHYTHMIAS, AND SUDDEN DEATH

Sudden death is defined as death occurring within 1-24 hr of collapse in a person with or without prior overt cardiac disease in whom there is no other probable cause of death. In witnessed deaths (in-hospital or out-of-hospital) the most common arrhythmia is ventricular fibrillation [1].

Sudden death represents a major source of cardiovascular mortality in the United States. It has been estimated that some 300,000 persons die in this manner every year [2]. Most have coronary artery disease and many have not had *any* prior clinical evidence of heart disease.

The Framingham Study has analyzed the risk factors for this phenomenon in 5209 persons and found that the "classical" risk factors of coronary artery disease appear to be risk factors for sudden death as well, especially in men [2]. Pathologic studies at necropsy have revealed several differences between those patients who were previously asymptomatic compared to those patients who had histories of angina pectoris and/or a clinical acute myocardial infarction [3]. In one study, peak age was 41-60 (Figure 1) and men predominated. There was a higher frequency of left main disease and a lower frequency of one-vessel disease in the symptomatic group. Quantitative analysis showed a significantly higher mean percent of severely narrowed segments in the symptomatic group and less minimal narrowing (Figure 2).

The degree of vascular pathology not withstanding, the intriguing question is whether patients with silent myocardial ischemia are as likely—or more likely—to develop sudden death than their symptomatic counterparts. In the absence of an effective anginal warning system [4], will individuals at high risk because of severe coronary stenoses continue to exert themselves until catastrophic events (sudden death or myocardial infarction) occur?

It is obvious that the widespread and extensive coronary atherosclerosis present at autopsy in individuals dying suddenly and unexpectedly did not occur overnight (although complete occlusion due to a thrombus—when present—is presumably a sudden event). Few studies have addressed the issue of whether the population with asymptomatic coronary artery disease

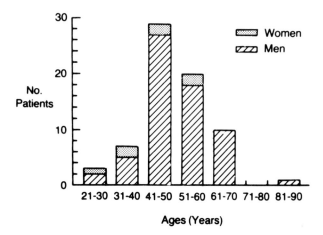

Figure 1   Age distribution in 70 patients with sudden coronary death. (From C. A. Warnes and W. C. Roberts. *Am. J. Cardiol.,* *54*:65, 1984.)

forms the pool from which a certain number of persons will surface each year as victims of sudden death or nonfatal myocardial infarctions. Evidence from a study performed at the Hennepin County Medical Center in Minnesota [5] provides some tentative conclusions in this regard. These investigators studied 15 persons who were successfully resuscitated from ventricular fibrillation that took place outside the hospital. Nine of the 15 had no prior history of heart disease. During bicycle exercise testing in the catheterization laboratory, nearly all the patients developed silent myocardial ischemia on their ECGs. Ventriculography also showed painless wall motion abnormalities (Figure 3). The severity of left ventricular dysfunction was similar in asymptomatic compared to the previously symptomatic patients. Thus, one could speculate that silent ischemia may have occurred prior to the episode of ventricular fibrillation and may play a role in the genesis of sudden death in some individuals.

Poole et al. [6], in a preliminary report, found that 25% of 43 out-of-hospital survivors of ventricular fibrillation had silent ischemia on Holter monitoring. Kattus at UCLA (personal communication) studied five previously asymptomatic coronary patients who were resuscitated from sudden death and demonstrated silent ischemia on exercise testing. Myerburg at the University of Miami (personal communication) has had a similar experience with three patients. Hong et al. [7] were able to document life-

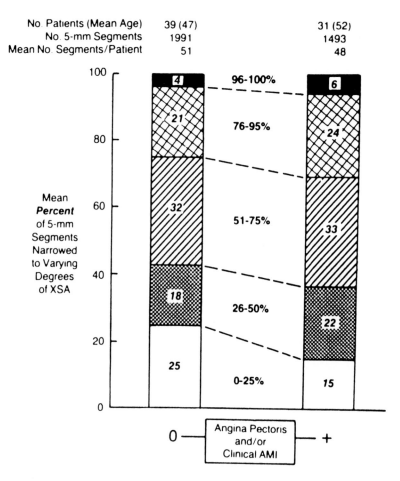

Figure 2 Mean percent of 5-mm segments of the sum of the four major coronary arteries narrowed to varying degrees in cross-sectional area (XSA) in 70 patients with sudden coronary death: comparison of 39 patients without and 31 patients with a clinical acute myocardial infarction (AMI) or angina or both. (From C. A. Warnes and W. C. Roberts. *Am. J. Cardiol., 54*:65, 1984.)

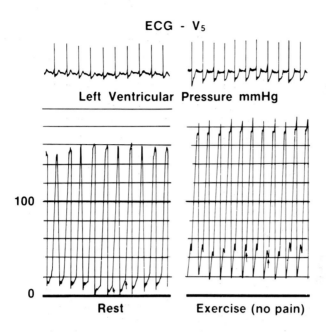

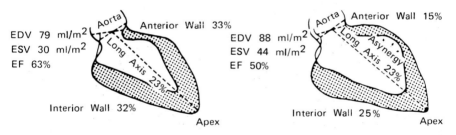

Left Ventriculogram

Figure 3 Simultaneous recording of chest lead V₅, left ventricular pressure and ventriculogram during exercise indicating electrocardiographic (ECG), hemodynamic and left ventriculographic evidence of painless myocardial ischemia in an asymptomatic patient with out-of-hospital ventricular fibrillation (patient 3). Note the increase in end-diastolic pressure from rest to exercise (arrows). EDV = end-diastolic volume; EF = ejection fraction; ESV = end-systolic volume. (From B. Sharma, R. Asinger, G. S. Francis, M. Hodges, and R. P. Wyeth. *Am. J. Cardiol., 59*:740, 1987.)

threatening ventricular arrhymias induced by silent ischemia on exercise tests in three patients. Meissner and Morganroth [8] reviewed records of patients dying during Holter monitoring. They concluded that many of the terminal events (perhaps as much as 25%) could represent ischemia-related deaths. Hohnloser et al. [9] report striking examples of this phenomenon in two patients. Despite these reports, the arrhythmogenic potential of silent ischemia—or any ischemic event for that matter—is still controversial [10,11]. Nonetheless, in Erikssen's study in Norway [12], 3 of 50 totally asymptomatic persons died suddenly and unexpectedly. Interestingly, seven others developed myocardial infarctions, of which two were silent. All three of the dead patients and six of the seven patients with myocardial infarctions had multivessel disease.

In the U.S. Air Force study, Hickman et al. [13] recorded two cases of sudden death (for an annual rate of 4.4/1000, while Feruglio [14] reported rates of 10/1000 in one series and 12/1000 in another series. This compares to rates of 2.9/1000 in epidemiologic studies using positive exercise tests without angiographic confirmation. By contrast, rates of 20-27/1000 for stable angina patients and 40-60/1000 for those with unstable angina have been reported (Table 1).

What implications do these data have in relation to vigorous exercise in asymptomatic individuals who may have latent coronary artery disease?

Table 1   Incidence of SD in Coronary Artery Disease

Patient category		Annual incidence (per 1000)
Symptomatic	Stable effort angina	20-27
	Unstable angina	40-60
	Acute myocardial infarction	$\geq 20\%$
	Previous infarction	50
Asymptomatic	No previous acute myocardial infarction	4.4 [16]
		2.9 [17]
		10 [8, 18]
	Previous myocardial infarction	12 [24]

SD = sudden death.
 Numbers in brackets indicate references in original article.
Source: G. A. Geruglio. In *Silent Myocardial Ischemia* (W. Rutishauser and H. Roskamm, eds.), Springer-Verlag, Berlin, 1984.

We know there is a small risk of sudden death in persons participating in vigorous sports. Northcote and Ballantyne reviewed the literature and found 109 such instances of which 80 (73%) were attributed to coronary artery disease found at autopsy [15]. They felt medical screening, including exercise testing, might be helpful in identifying some of the individuals at highest risk. They have been particularly interested in squash playing in the United Kingdom and in 1986 reported on 60 deaths occurring between 1976 and 1984 [16]. Only 22 of the persons had known medical conditions possibly related to heart disease, yet 51/60 had autopsy-proven coronary artery disease. Proximal symptoms were present in some but not all of the patients without known heart disease (Madsen [17]) has observed that about 20% of sudden death victims have neither prodromes nor overt heart disease). In contrast to the British experience, Malinow et al. found only one case of sudden death in a 10-year retrospective analysis of YMCA sports facilities in the United States [18]. Therefore, they felt it was not important to screen such persons. Siscovick et al. [19] interviewed the wives of 133 men without known prior heart disease who had suffered a cardiac arrest. They concluded that those persons who engaged in low levels of habitual physical activity had a greater risk of sudden death during vigorous exercise compared to more physically active men. Whether exercise ECG screening prior to performing vigorous activity would have detected latent coronary artery disease in these individuals is unclear [20].

II. SILENT MYOCARDIAL ISCHEMIA AND SILENT MYOCARDIAL INFARCTION

It is tempting to speculate that if myocardial infarction occurs—rather than sudden death—it is more likely to be silent in this group of individuals. Are there any data to support this conjecture? Only in Erikksen's study [12], where 2 of 50 asymptomatic patients with angiographically confirmed disease developed silent infarctions. Whether patients with both silent ischemia and angina tend to develop silent infarctions is also unclear, though one could speculate that this circumstance must be common, since 20-25% of all infarctions are unrecognized.

III. SILENT MYOCARDIAL ISCHEMIA AND ISCHEMIC CARDIOMYOPATHY

Ischemia of the myocardium can cause diffuse fibrosis with the resultant clinical syndrome being indistinguishable from that of a primary congestive cardiomyopathy. It has generally been assumed that these cases represent "burned out" postinfarction patients who no longer have ischemic foci. A history of angina is usually, but not invariably, present. However, in many cases there has been neither an anginal history nor a history of a symptomatic infarciton. Pantely and Bristow [21] speculate that "repeated episodes of silent ischemia, though brief, or silent infarction, though small, may result in congestive ischemic cardiomyopathy" in such patients. Presumably the mechanism would be similar to that of the "stunned" or "hibernating" myocardium described in Chapter 4. Raper et al. [22] in their small series of patients with severe painless ischemia offer dramatic evidence of how a painless episode can lead to marked left ventricular dysfunction, including pulmonary edema.

   Survival in patients with this syndrome—as in all types of cardiomyopathy—is directly related to the degree of left ventricular dysfunction.

IV. CONCLUSIONS

It is intriguing to speculate the silent myocardial ischemia can lead to sudden death, silent infarcts or even ischemic cardiomyopathy. There is evidence to confirm this sequence in some patients, but the numbers are too small to permit sweeping generalizations.

REFERENCES

1. S. Goldstein, L. Friedman, R. Hutchinson, P. Canner, D. Romhilt, R. Schlant, R. Sobrino, J. Verter, A. Wasserman, and the Aspirin Myocardial Infarction Study Research Group. Timing, mechanism and clinical setting of witnessed deaths in postmyocardial infarction patients. *J. Am. Coll. Cardiol., 3*:111 (1984).

2. A. Schatzkin, L. A. Cupples, T. Heeren, S. Morelock, M. Mucatel, and W. B. Kannel. The epidemiology of sudden unexpected death: Risk factors for men and women in the Framingham Heart Study. *Am. Heart J., 107*:1300 (1984).

3. C. A. Warnes and W. C. Roberts. Sudden coronary death: Relation of amount and distribution of coronary narrowing at necropsy to previous symptoms of myocardial ischemia, left ventricular scarring and heart weight. *Am. J. Cardiol., 54*:65 (1984).

4. P. F. Cohn. Silent myocardial ischemia in patients with a defective anginal warning system. *Am. J. Cardiol., 45*:697 (1980).

5. B. Sharma, R. Asinger, G. S. Francis, M. Hodges, and R. P. Wyeth. Demonstration of exercise-induced painless myocardial ischemia in survivors of out-of-hospital ventricular fibrillation. *Am. J. Cardiol., 59*:740 (1987).

6. B. Norris, D. B. Callahan, M. Emery, and L. A. Cobb. Silent ischemia in survivors of out-of-hospital ventricular fibrillation (abstr). *J. Am. Coll. Cardiol., 11*:96A (1988).

7. R. A. Hong, A. K. Bhandari, C. R. McKay, P. K. Au, and S. H. Rahimtoola. Life-threatening ventricular tachycardia and fibrillation induced by painless myocardial ischemia during exercise testing. *J.A.M.A., 257*:1937 (1987).

8. M. D. Meissner and J. Morganroth. Silent myocardial ischemia as a mechanism of sudden death. *Cardiol. Clin., 4*(4):593 (1986).

9. S. H. Hohnloser, W. Kasper, M. Zehender, A. Geibel, T. Meinertz, and H. Just. Silent myocardial ischemia as a predisposing factor for ventricular fibrillation. *Am. J. Cardiol., 61*:461 (1988).

10. P. Mathes, A. Reinke, and D. Michel. Arrhythmogenic potential of silent myocardial ischemia after myocardial infarction. In *Silent Ischemia: Current Concepts and Management* (T. von Arnim and A. Maseri, eds.), Steinkopff, Darmstadt, 1987, p. 56-61.

11. J. A. Gomes, D. Alexopoulos, S. Winters, V. Fuster, and K. Suh. The role of silent ischemia and the electrophysiologic substrate in the genesis of sudden cardiac death (abstr). *J. Am. Coll. Cardiol., 11*:6A (1988).

12. J. Erikssen and E. Thaulow. Follow-up of patients with asymptomatic myocardial ischemia. In *Silent Myocardial Ischemia* (W. Rutishauser and H. Roskamm, eds.), Springer-Verlag, Berlin, 1984, pp. 156-164.

13. J. R. Hickman, Jr., G. S. Uhl, R. L. Cook, P. J. Engel, and A. Hopkirk. A natural study of asymptomatic coronary disease (abstr). *Am. J. Cardiol., 45*: 422 (1980).

14. G. A. Feruglio. Sudden death in patients with asymptomatic coronary heart disease. In *Silent Myocardial Ischemia* (W. Rutishauser and H. Roskamm, eds.), Springer-Verlag, Berlin, 1984, pp. 144-150.

15. R. J. Northcote and D. Ballantyne. Sudden cardiac death in sport. *Br. Med. J., 287*:1357 (1983).

16. R. J. Northcote, C. Flannigan, and D. Ballantyne. Sudden death and vigorous exercise—A study of 60 deaths associated with squash. *Br. Heart J., 55*: 198 (1986).

17. J. K. Madsen. Ischaemic heart disease and prodromes of sudden cardiac death: Is it possible to identify high risk groups for sudden cardiac death? *Br. Heart J., 54*:27 (1985).

18. M. R. Malinow, D. L. McGarry, and K. S. Kuehl. Is exercise testing indicated for asymptomatic active people? *J. Cardiac Rehabil., 4*:376 (1984).

19. D. S. Siscovick, N. S. Weiss, R. H. Fletcher, and T. Lasky. Relation between vigorous exercise and primary cardiac arrest. *N. Engl. J. Med., 311*:874 (1984).

20. P. F. Cohn. Silent myocardial ischemia: Clinical significance and relation to sudden cardiac death. *Chest, 90*:597 (1986).

21. G. A. Pantely and J. D. Bristow. Ischemic cardiomyopathy. *Prog. Cardio-vasc. Dis., 27*:95 (1984).

22. A. J. Raper, A. Hastillo, and W. J. Paulsen. The syndrome of sudden severe painless myocardial ischemia. *Am. Heart J., 107*:813 (1984).

14

Prognosis After Silent Myocardial Infarction and Myocardial Infarction Without Preceding Angina

Cardiologists have long appreciated that the natural history of coronary artery disease is complex because of the numerous "subsets" of patients with or without angina, with or without infarctions, etc. [1]. Unfortunately, data on prognosis following silent infarctions are sparse. The greatest source of data concerning this subset of patients has been the Framingham Study.

I. SILENT MYOCARDIAL INFARCTION

The Framingham survey was begun in 1948. A standard, thorough, cardiovascular examination was done biennially to detect newly developed cardiovascular disease. In addition, data on cardiovascular endpoints was also obtained by daily surveillance of hospital admission records at Framingham Union Hospital.

As discussed in Chapter 5, the myocardial infarctions were designated as "unrecognized" and then further subdivided into atypical or silent, depending on whether the patients—in retrospect—could identify any complaints as having possibly been compatible with an acute myocardial infarction. (About half of the 108 infarctions were of the truly silent type.) As reported in the 20-year follow-up, the 3-year mortality rates for both unrecognized and recognized myocardial infarctions were similar [2]. (In the Israeli study of Medalie and Goldbourt [3], the mortality following unrecognized myocardial infarctions was markedly lower than after recognized myocardial infarctions—unlike the Framingham experience.)

In their most recent report (26-year follow-up), the Framingham investigators have updated their results (4,5). As before, there are no data

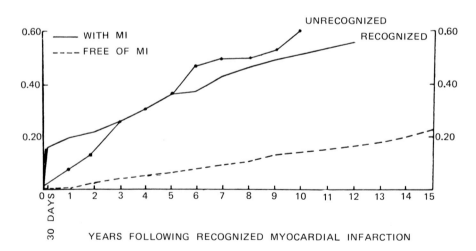

Figure 1 Death following recognized and unrecognized myocardial infarctions (MI) in men of all ages in the Framingham Study. (From W. B. Kannel and R. D. Abbott. In *Silent Myocardial Ischemia.* _____ = with MI; - - - = free of MI. [W. Rutishauser and H. Roskamm, eds.), Springer-Verlag, Berlin, 1984, pp. 131-137.)

Table 1 Proportion of ECG-Documented Myocardial Infarctions (MI) Followed by Angina Pectoris (AP) in Subjects Aged 30-62 Years on Entry. Framingham Study, 22-Year Follow-up

	Number with MI	Followed by AP	
		n	%
Unrecognized	98	18	18
Recognized	190	113	59
Total	288	114	45

Eighty-nine patients had prior angina pectoris or died and were eliminated from consideration.
Source: W. B. Kannel and R. D. Abbott. In *Silent Myocardial Ischemia* (W. Rutishauser and H. Roskamm, eds.), Springer-Verlag, Berlin, 1984, pp. 131-137.

Table 2 Proportion of ECG-Documented Myocardial Infarctions Followed by Cardiac Failure in Subjects 30-62 Years of Age at Entry. Framingham Study, 22-Year Follow-up

	Number	Followed by cardiac failure	
		n	%
Unrecognized	100	21	21
Recognized	221	55	25
Total	321	76	24

Source: W. B. Kannel and R. D. Abbott. In *Silent Myocardial Ischemia* (W. Rutishauser and H. Roskamm, eds.), Springer-Verlag, Berlin, 1984, pp. 131-137.

available on prognosis in the immediate convalescent period since, by definition, these patients are not identified until the next routine ECG is performed. However, in those who survived the initial period, the mortality statistics are sobering. As depicted in Figure 1, unrecognized infarctions are as potentially lethal as the symptomatic kind. After 10 years, 45% of patients with unrecognized and 39% of those with recognized infarctions were dead. Sudden deaths occurred with equal frequency, and at about nine times the rate seen in the general population. Although less prone to angina (18% vs. 59%) (Table 1), patients with unrecognized infarctions develop congestive heart failure just as often (Table 2). Reinfarction is also common (3%/year in men and 10%/year in women). About 50% of the recurrences are fatal. In the elderly population in the Framingham study, patients with recognized and unrecognized infarctions also had similar mortality rates [6].

Silent infarction can also be followed by silent ischemia either on the exercise test, Holter monitoring, or both [7].

II. MYOCARDIAL INFARCTION WITHOUT PRECEDING ANGINA

In patients who survive an acute myocardial infarction, about half did not have angina pectoris before the infarction [8-10]. As noted previously in Chapter 5, there is a high association of one-vessel disease (82%) in such patients [11]. One would suspect that prognosis might, therefore, be better in this type of patient and indeed Midwall et al. [11] reported a lower frequency of postinfarction angina. Mortality figures were not available in this study, but they were in the study by Pierard et al. [10]: 3-year mortality was 16% (angina) vs. 7% (no angina). This was similar to what Harper et al. [8] had reported in their series; hospital mortality was 12% in patients without preceding angina compared to 20% in patients with chronic stable angina. Long-term mortality statistics were also not available in this study. A recent study by Matsuda et al. [12] suggests that postinfarction left ventricular function is better in patients with angina and an occluded left anterior descending coronary artery compared to those with a similar lesion but without angina. No ready explanation for this finding is available, though the authors suggest better developed collaterals may be involved. Cortina et al. [13] reported similar findings.

III. CONCLUSIONS

Silent myocardial infarctions are as potentially lethal as the symptomatic kind. When a symptomatic infarction occurs, prognosis is better if the patient did not have angina preceding the infarction.

REFERENCES

1. G. J. Goldman and A. D. Pichard. The natural history of coronary artery disease: Does medical therapy improve the prognosis? *Prog. Cardiovasc. Dis., 25*: 513 (1983).

2. W. B. Kannel, P. Sorlie, and P. M. McNamara. Prognosis after initial myocardial infarction: The Framingham Study. *Am. J. Cardiol., 44*:53 (1979).

3. J. H. Medalie and M. A. Goldbourt. Unrecognized myocardial infarction: Five-year incidence, mortality and risk factors. *Ann. Intern. Med., 84*:526 (1976).

4. W. B. Kannel and R. D. Abbott. Incidence and prognosis of unrecognized myocardial infarction: Based on 26 years follow-up in the Framingham Study. In *Silent Myocardial Ischemia* (W. Rutishauser and H. Roskamm, eds.), Springer-Verlag, Berlin, 1984, pp. 131-137.

5. W. B. Kannel and R. D. Abbott. Incidence and prognosis of unrecognized myocardial infarction. An update on the Framingham Study. *N. Engl. J. Med., 311*:1144 (1984).

6. P. S. Vokonas, W. B. Kannel, and L. A. Cupples. Incidence and prognosis of unrecognized myocardial infarction in the elderly, The Framingham Study (abstr). *J. Am. Coll. Cardiol., 11*:51A, 1988.

7. P. F. Cohn, M. T. Sodums, W. E. Lawson, S. C. Vlay, and E. J. Brown, Jr. Frequent episodes of silent myocardial ischemia after apparently uncomplicated myocardial infarction. *J. Am. Coll. Cardiol., 8*:982 (1986).

8. R. W. Harper, G. Kennedy, R. W. DeSanctis, and A. M. Hutter, Jr. The incidence and pattern of angina prior to acute myocardial infarction: A study of 577 cases. *Am. Heart J., 97*:178 (1979).

9. M. Matsuda, Y. Matsuda, H. Ogawa, K. Moritani, and R. Kusukawa. Angina pectoris before and during acute myocardial infarction: Relation to degree of physical activity. *Am. J. Cardiol., 55*:1255 (1985).

10. L. A. Pierard, C. Dubois, J-P. Smeets, J. Boland, J. Carlier, and H. E. Kulbertus. Prognostic significance of angina pectoris before first acute myocardial infarction. *Am. J. Cardiol., 61*:984 (1988).

11. J. Midwall, J. Ambrose, A. Pichard, Z. Abedin, and M. V. Herman. Angina pectoris before and after myocardial infarction: angiographic correlations. *Chest, 81*:681 (1982).

12. Y. Matsuda, H. Ogawa, K. Moritani, M. Matsuda, H. Naito, M. Matsuzaki, Y. Ikee, and R. Kusukawa. Effects of the presence or absence of preceding angina pectoris on left ventricular function after acute myocardial infarction. *Am. Heart J., 108*:955 (1984).

13. A. Cortina, J. A. Ambrose, J. Prieto-Granada, C. Moris, E. Simarro, J. Holt, and V. Fuster. Left ventricular function after myocardial infarction: Clinical and angiographic correlations. *J. Am. Coll. Cardiol., 5*:619 (1985).

V
MANAGEMENT OF PATIENTS WITH ASYMPTOMATIC CORONARY ARTERY DISEASE

15

Medical Treatment of Asymptomatic Coronary Artery Disease

Having diagnosed patients as having silent ischemia, the physician must then decide on appropriate therapy—if he chooses to treat at all. Guidelines can be offered on the basis of the prognostic information provided in the preceding section, as well as the results of pilot studies and other therapeutic trials that are completed or still underway [1-3].

I. MANAGEMENT OF PERSONS WHO ARE TOTALLY ASYMPTOMATIC

Perhaps no single area concerning asymptomatic coronary artery disease is as controversial as management [4]. Because the prognosis in persons in this category is generally favorable, the simplest approach is to (1) modify risk factors when they are present and (2) reduce physical activities so that myocardial ischemia does not develop. The latter is to ward off possible damage to the patient with a defective angina warning system during strenuous exertion. It is the patients who demonstrate extensive ischemia that merit special concern [4]. These individuals are more likely to have multivessel disease with its correspondingly worse prognosis. As opposed to asymptomatic persons with single-vessel disease who may be in a "presymptomatic" stage and go on to angina or nonfatal infarction, asymptomatic individuals with triple-vessel or left main disease appear to be at higher risk for sudden death or massive infarctions. We believe every effort should be made to treat these latter patients with antiischemic agents. One endpoint could be improved exercise tolerance, i.e., prolonging the time at which ischemia develops. Another endpoint could be improved wall motion in ischemic zones. This can be documented in one of several ways. For example, in a pilot study from our laboratory [5], we treated eleven asymptomatic patients with silent myocardial ischemia (some of whom had prior infarctions) with propranolol or timolol and evaluated exercise ECGs and radionuclide ventriculograms before and after administration of the drugs. The beneficial results are depicted in Table 1. Whether prognosis is improved in these patients cannot be proven at present. Another way to approach the asymptomatic patient with silent ischemia is to

Table 1 Treatment of Silent Myocardial Ischemia with Beta-Adrenergic Blockage (BAB)

	Pre-BAB	Post-BAB	p value
Time to exercise- induced ST depression	207 sec $\pm$ 75	348 sec $\pm$ 89	$p < 0.05$
Maximum ST depression	1.41 mm $\pm$ 0.15	0.81 $\pm$ 0.20	$p < 0.05$
Change in regional exercise ejection fraction	-0.06 ± 0.01	-0.01 ± 0.01	$p < 0.01$

use Holter monitoring to document a reduction in ischemic activity (either frequency, duration, or both). Imperi et al. [6] used the beta blocker metoprolol in a group of nine asymptomatic or minimally symptomatic patients. By titrating the metoprolol to an optimal dose (via Holter monitoring), they were able to significantly reduce ischemic activity. We achieved similar results (Table 2) using the calcium blocker nifedipine in a standard dose, either 30 or 60 mg daily [7].

Although usually employed in symptomatic patients, percutaneous transluminal coronary angioplasty (PTCA) can be used in selected asymptomatic patients [8].

Because psychological stress may exacerbate silent myocardial ischemia [9], psychological counseling is important in these patients, especially since the implications of a potentially lethal but silent disease can be further anxiety-provoking and thus detrimental to the patient's emotional well-being [10]. This is discussed further in the following section on postinfarction patients.

Table 2 Clinical, Angiographic, and Holter Findings Before and After Nifedipine in 12 Asymptomatic Patients

				Holter monitoring			
				Pretreatment		Nifedipine treatment	
	Narrowed CA			Ischemic episodes (n)	Duration of ischemic episodes (min)	Ischemic episodes (n)	Duration of ischemic episodes (min)
Pt	Right	LAD	LC	MI			
1	+	+	+	0	11	699	4	143
2	+	0	0	0	6	153	4	144
3	+	+	0	+(A)	4	15	1	2
4	0	+	+	+(A)	6	53	1	10
5	+	+	+	0	3	39	4	21
6	+	+	+	+(I)	17	120	5	59
7	+	0	0	0	4	14	1	2
8	+	+	0	0	8	40	0	0
9	+	+	+	0	6	37	6	55
10	0	+	0	0	4	197	7	177
11	+	+	+	+(A)	5	52	0	0
12	+	+	+	0	6	68	4	2

A = anterior; CA = coronary artery; I = inferior; LAD = left anterior descending coronary artery; LC = left circumflex coronary artery; MI = myocardial infarction.
Source: P. F. Cohn and W. E. Lawson. *Am. J. Cardiol., 61*:908, 1988.

II. MANAGEMENT OF PATIENTS WHO ARE ASYMPTOMATIC FOLLOWING A MYOCARDIAL INFARCTION

There is a greater consensus concerning treatment of these patients. Even those who are skeptical of treating totally asymptomatic persons would treat postinfarction patients with silent ischemia [11]. At present, medical treatment with beta blockers is recommended for postinfarction patients in order to reduce short-term mortality and reinfarction [12]. Therefore, it is only logical that *all* patients with evidence of myocardial ischemia postinfarction should receive some form of medical treatment, whether or not they are symptomatic.

As discussed previously in Chapter 11, most physicians regard continuing evidence of ischemia as grounds for cardiac catheterization. Depending on the severity of the angiographic findings, some of these patients will be candidates for more aggressive medical management, coronary angioplasty, or coronary bypass surgery. Comparisons of medical versus surgical management (as in the CASS survey) will be discussed in the next chapter.

Psychological reactions in these patients are also important, since many assume that once they have recovered from the acute infarction and are asymptomatic, they have little to worry about. When this assumption is corrected, the level of anxiety is raised. However in a study of 15 patients [10] with asymptomatic coronary artery disease, most of whom had prior infarctions, we found that most patients felt their physicians had been supportive in explaining the problems to them. Because of trust in their physicians, patients often changed their lifestyles markedly in regard to exercise and diet. All agreed that public awareness of this disorder was unfortunately almost nonexistent.

III. MANAGEMENT OF PATIENTS WITH EPISODES OF BOTH SYMPTOMATIC AND ASYMPTOMATIC MYOCARDIAL ISCHEMIA

These patients are the ones that practitioners are most likely to encounter. In the past, there has been a tendency to discount the importance of the asymptomatic episodes and to treat "symptoms." With the report of several groups that asymptomatic episodes often greatly outnumber symptomatic episodes (as determined by Holter monitoring), there is a growing trend toward considering the asymptomatic episodes of equal importance to the symptomatic ones. Both can result in metabolic, hemodynamic and electrical abnormalities of myocardial function. As a result, a new approach to the treatment of myocardial ischemia is gaining acceptance. In this approach, the use of drugs, angioplasty, and surgery is used to reduce the *total ischemic burden* and not merely symptomatic episodes [1,13]. (One group has reported that the greatest number of ischemic episodes per day appears to be in those patients with both symptomatic and painless ischemia [14]).

Just as with Type 1 and Type 2 patients discussed earlier, choice of medications in Type 3 patients depends on whether the ischemia is due to increased work of the heart or to a vasospastic component or both. In the former case, myocardial oxygen requirements are raised, usually because of increases in heart rate and blood pressure, two of the major factors regulating myocardial oxygen consumption. For these episodes, beta-blockers would appear to be reasonable agents.

However, many of the episodes do *not* appear to be associated with increased work of the heart. For example, Schang and Pepine [15] and the more recently Cecchi et al. (Figure 1) [16] reported that the ratio of asymptomatic episodes to symptomatic episodes recorded on Holter monitoring was greatest during nonstrenuous activities. This suggests a role for increased vasoconstrictor tone. Further evidence is provided by the lack of increased heart rate or blood pressure preceding many episodes, as in the example in Figure 2, from the study of hospitalized patients by Chierchia et al. [17]. Ambulatory blood pressure records in out-of-hospital patients have shown similar results [18]. Furthermore, Deanfield et al. [19] demonstrated that in their patients the heart rate at the onset of ST segment depression was significantly lower after unprovoked ischemia than after exercise (Figure 3). Peak heart rates showed the same trend. During silent myocardial ischemia due to mental stress, heart rate was also less than during exercise-induced ischemia. It would, therefore, seem reasonable that for episodes of silent ischemia not associated with increased work of the heart, nitrates or calcium antagonists would provide the best approach to therapy. Schang and Pepine [15] were able to significantly reduce the frequency of asymptomatic episodes using hourly nitroglycerin tablets (3.7 ± 0.02 episodes per monitoring period to 0.6 ± 0.02). Johnson et al. [20] and Parodi et al. [21] reduced total ischemic episodes with verapamil. Frishman et al. did the same with diltiazem. In a small series of patients, Oakley et al. [23] used nifedipine with good results—though best results were observed when nifedipine and propranolol were combined. The combination of nifedipine and beta-blockers has also been used in the Nifedipine-Total Ischemia Awareness Program (TIAP) [3].

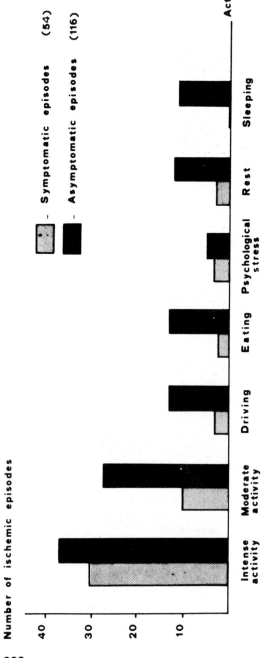

Figure 1 Activity at the onset of ischemic attacks. Intense physical activity—jogging, playing tennis, bicycling, walking upstairs, and sexual activity. Moderate physical activity—slow walking, light housework, and light hand labor. (From A. C. Cecchi, E. V. Dovellini, F. Marchi, P. Pucci, C. M. Santoro, and P. F. Fazzini. *J. Am. Coll. Cardiol., 1*:934, 1983.)

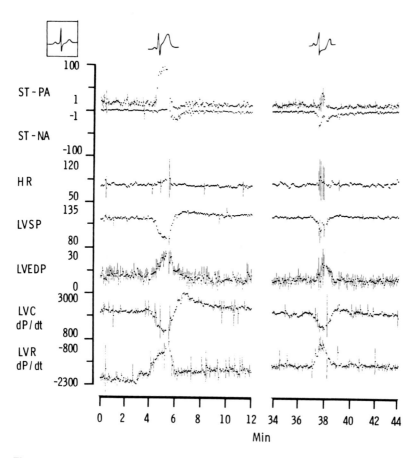

Figure 2 Computer plot of two asymptomatic ischemic episodes in the same patient. The averaged values of each derived variable are plotted with their standard deviation against time. The variables (top to bottom) were ST segment positive (PA) and negative areas (NA), heart rate (HR), left ventricular systolic (LVSP) and end-diastolic pressures (LVEDP) and left ventricular peak contraction (LVC) and relaxation (LVR) dP/dt. In the episode on the left, transient ST segment elevation (increase in ST segment positive area) was accompanied by an increase in left ventricular end-diastolic pressure, and decreases in both contract and relaxation dP/dt. Similar impairment of left ventricular function accompanied the asymptomatic episode of ST segment depression (increase in ST segment negative area) in the same electrocardiographic lead shown on the right. A vasospastic component is suggested by the lack of increase in the variables controlling myocardial oxygen demand (such as HR or LVSP) before either episode. (From S. Cherichia, M. Lazzari, B. Freedman, C. Brunelli, and A. Maseri. *J. Am. Coll. Cardiol., 1*:924, 1983.)

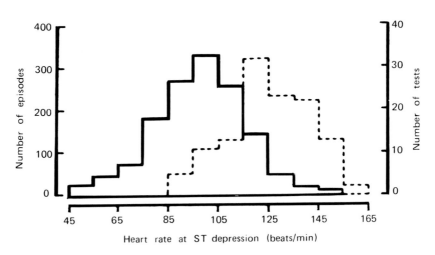

Figure 3 Distribution of heart rates at onset of ST depression during ambulatory monitoring (_____) and during exercise testing (- - -). (From J. E. Deanfield, A. P. Selwyn, S. Krikler, and M. Morgan. *Lancet, 2*:753, 1983.)

Nifedipine led to a further and significant reduction in ischemic activity when added to either nitrates and/or beta-blockers. The beneficial effects of combination therapy were especially marked in the patients with the most total ischemic activity (Table 3).

Table 3 Effect of Nifedipine on Number and Duration of Silent Ischemic Episodes in 38 Patients in the Total Ischemia Awareness Program (TIAP) with 60 Minutes or More of Ischemic Activity While Taking Nitrates and/or Beta Blockers for Angina

	Pre-Nifedipine (mean ± SEM)	Post-Nifedipine (mean ± SEM)
ST segment changes without pain (no.)	5.7 ± 0.9	3.2 ± 0.6, $p < 0.001$
Depressed ST segment duration (min.)	127 ± 13	68 ± 15, $p < 0.001$

Table 4 Effect of Transdermal Nitroglycerin on Number and Duration of Ischemic Events in Eight Patients with Chronic Angina

	Pre-Nitroglycerin (mean ± SEM)	Post-Nitroglycerin (mean ± SEM)
Silent ischemic episodes (no.)	5.3 ± 3.3	0.8 ± 1.2 ($p < 0.05$)
Depressed ST segment duration (min.)	95.8 ± 87	17 ± 27.1 ($p = 0.05$)

Source: Adapted from W. E. Shell, C. F. Kivowitz, S. B. Rubins, and J. See. *Am. Heart J., 212*:222, 1986.

Despite the observations concerning relatively low heart rates at the onset of most episodes of out-of-hospital ischemia and their lack of association with strenuous exertion, the beta blockers have also been useful in reducing ischemic activity on Holter recordings. In addition to the metoprolol studies [6,24], there have been favorable responses with propranolol [25] and atenolol [26]. Long-acting nitrates [27,28] have also proven efficacious (Table 4). Silent ischemia has also been abolished after coronary angioplasty [29] (Figure 4). By contrast, persistent silent ischemia following angioplasty has been associated with an increased incidence of cardiac events [30]. Only one trial of aspirin has been reported, and that was without success. Whether this was because of dosage or other factors is not clear, but the study deserves to be repeated in light of speculation concerning the role of enhanced platelet aggregability in causing ischemic events.

IV. MANAGEMENT OF SILENT MYOCARDIAL INFARCTION

Recognition of these events invariably occurs too late for the usual treatment accorded patients with infarctions. However, patients at times may present with the acute *complications* of a silent infarction and require appropriate management. An example is the patient in pulmonary edema reported by Raper et al. [31].

V. CONCLUSIONS

Medical management of silent myocardial ischemia involves modification or risk factors, use of drugs and in, appropriate patients, angioplasty. Although beta-blockade appears efficacious (especially during exertion),

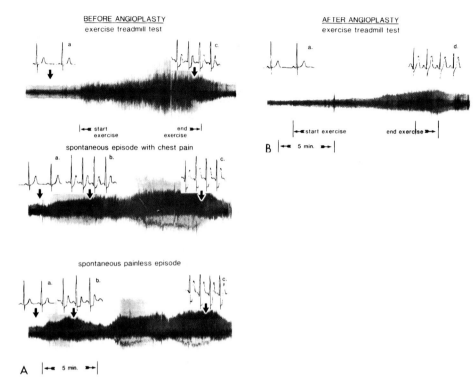

Figure 4 (*A*) Selected portions of the 24-hr Holter compact analog record before angioplasty in a patient with an 80% stenosis in the proximal portion of the left anterior descending coronary artery. The *upper panel* was recorded during treadmill exercise test, the *middle panel* during a spontaneous episode of angina and the *lower panel* during a spontaneous episode of ischemia without associated chest pain. The inserted printouts at a paper speed of 25 mm/sec demonstrate the normal QRST complex (a), ST segment depression at the onset of ischemia (b), and marked ST segment depression with T wave augmentation (c). The ST segment depression and T wave augmentation during spontaneous episodes of ischemia are similar to those induced during exercise. (*B*) After angioplasty, only T wave augmentation without ST segment depression (d) occurred at 13.2 min of treadmill exercise. No spontaneous episodes were present on the Holter recording in this patient after angioplasty. (From M. A. Josephson, K. Nademanee, V. Intarachot, H. Lewis, and B. N. Singh. *J. Am. Coll. Cardiol., 10*:499, 1987.)

many of the ischemic episodes appear to have a vasospastic component, suggesting that calcium antagonists and nitrates may also be useful. In evaluating any drug, however, the natural variability of ischemic events must be considered [32,33].

REFERENCES

1. C. J. Pepine, G. A. Imperi, and J. A. Hill. Therapeutic implications of silent myocardial ischemia during daily activity. *Am. J. Cardiol., 59*:993 (1987).

2. W. H. Frishman and M. Teicher. Antianginal drug therapy for silent myocardial ischemia. *Am. Heart J., 114*:140 (1987).

3. P. F. Cohn, G. W. Vetrovec, R. Nesto, and the Total Ischemia Awareness Program Investigators. The Nifedipine-Total Ischemia Awareness Program: A national survey of painful and painless myocardial ischemia including results of anti-ischemic therapy. *Am. J. Cardiol.* (in press, March 1989).

4. P. F. Cohn, E. J. Brown, Jr., and J. K. Cohn. Detection and management of coronary artery disease in the asymptomatic population. *Am. Heart J., 108*:1064 (1984).

5. P. F. Cohn, E. J. Brown, Jr., Rita Swinford, and H. L. Atkins. Effect of beta blockade on silent regional left ventricular wall motion abnormalities. *Am. J. Cardiol., 57*:521 (1986).

6. G. A. Imperi, C. R. Lambert, K. Coy, L. Lopez, and C. J. Pepine. Effects of titrated beta blockade (metoprolol) on silent myocardial ischemia in ambulatory patients with coronary artery disease. *Am. J. Cardiol., 60*:519 (1987).

7. P. F. Cohn and W. E. Lawson. Effect of nifedipine on out-of-hospital silent myocardial ischemia in asymptomatic men with coronary artery disease. *Am. J. Cardiol., 61*:908 (1988).

8. K. M. Kent. Transluminal coronary angioplasty in asymptomatic or mildly symptomatic patients. *Circulation, 75*(Suppl II):45 (1987).

9. L. J. Freeman, P. G. F. Nixon, P. Sallabank, and D. Reaveley. Psychological stress and silent myocardial ischemia. *Am. Heart J., 114*:477 (1987).

10. J. K. Cohn and P. F. Cohn. Patient reactions to the diagnosis of asymptomatic coronary artery disease: Implications for the primary physician and consultant cardiologist. *J. Am. Coll. Cardiol., 1*:956 (1983).

11. R. F. Leighton and T. D. Fraker, Jr. Silent myocardial ischemia: Concern is justified for the patient with known coronary artery disease. *Ann. Intern. Med., 100*:599 (1984).

12. L. Goldman, S. T. B. Sia, E. F. Cook, J. D. Rutherford, and M. C. Weinstein. Costs and effectiveness of routine therapy with long-term beta-adrenergic antagonnists after acute myocardial infarction. *N. Engl. J. Med., 319*:152 (1988).

13. P. F. Cohn. Time for a new approach to the management of patients with both symptomatic and asymptomatic episodes of myocardial ischemia. *Am. J. Cardiol., 54*:1357 (1984).

14. S. Stern, A. Gavish, G. Weisz, J. Benhorin, A. Keren, and D. Tzivoni. Characteristics of silent and symptomatic myocardial ischemia during daily activities. *Am. J. Cardiol., 61*:1223 (1988).

15. J. J. Schang, Jr., and C. J. Pepine. Transient asymptomatic ST-segment depression during daily activity. *Am. J. Cardiol., 39*:396 (1977).

16. A. C. Cecchi, E. V. Dovellini, F. Marchi, P. Pucci, C. M. Santoro, and P. F. Fazzini. Silent myocardial ischemia during ambulatory electrocardiographic monitoring in patients with effort angina. *J. Am. Coll. Cardiol., 1*:934 (1983).

17. S. Chierchia, M. Lazzari, B. Freedman, C. Brunelli, and A. Maseri. Impairment of myocardial perfusion and function during painless myocardial ischemia. *J. Am. Coll. Cardiol., 1*:924 (1983).

18. M. H. Crawford, J. Vittitoe, and R. A. O'Rourke. Ambulatory blood pressure recordings during silent ischemia episodes (abstr). *Circulation, 76*(Suppl IV):79 (1987).

19. J. E. Deanfield, M. Shea, P. Ribiero, C. M. deLandsheere, R. A. Wilson, P. Horlock, and A. P. Selwyn. Transient ST segment depression as a marker of myocardial ischemia during daily life: A physiological validation in patients with angina and coronary disease. *Am. J. Cardiol., 54*:1195 (1984).

20. S. M. Johnson, D. R. Mauritson, J. T. Willerson, and L. D. Hillis. A controlled trial of verapamil for Prinzmetal's variant angina. *N. Engl. J. Med., 304*:862 (1981).

21. O. Parodi, I. Simonetii, C. Michelassi, C. Carpeggiani, A. Biagini, A. L'Abbate, and A. Maseri. Comparison of verapamil and propranolol therapy for angina pectoris at rest: A randomized, multiple-crossover, controlled trial in the coronary care unit. *Am. J. Cardiol., 57*:899 (1986).

22. G. D. G. Oakley, K. M. Fox, H. J. Dargie, and A. P. Selwyn. Objective assessment of therapy in severe angina. *Br. Med. J., 1*:1540 (1979).

23. K. Egstrup. Randomized double-blind comparison of metoprolol, nifedipine, and their combination in chronic stable angina: Effects on total ischemic activity and heart rate at onset of ischemia. *Am. Heart J. 116*:971 (1988).

24. W. Frishman, S. Charlap, B. Kimmel, M. Teicher, J. Cinnamon, L. Allen, and J. Strom. Diltiazem, nifedipine and their combination in patients with stable angina pectoris: Effects on angina, exercise tolerance and the ambulatory electrocardiographic ST segment. *Circulation, 77*:774 (1988).

25. D. T. Kawanishi, C. L. Reid, G. Simsarian, Y. Amisola, A. Gonzales, and S. H. Rahimtoola. Effect of pharmacologic therapy on angina frequency, ST segment depression during ambulatory ECG monitoring, and treadmill per-

formance in patients with chronic stable mild angina. *Am. Heart J., 115*:220 (1988).

26. A. A. Quyyumi, T. Crake, C. M. Wright, L. J. Mockus, and K. M. Fox. Medical treatment of patients with severe exertinal and rest angina: double blind comparison of blocker, calcium antagonist, and nitrate. *Br. Heart J., 57*:505 (1987).

27. W. E. Shell, C. F. Kivowitz, S. B. Rubins, and J. See. Mechanisms and therapy of silent myocardial ischemia: The effect of transdermal nitroglycerin. *Am. Heart J., 212*:222 (1986).

28. T. vonArnim and A. Erath. Nitrates and calcium antagonists for silent myocardial ischemia. *Am. J. Cardiol., 61*:15E (1988).

29. M. A. Josephson, K. Nademanee, V. Intarachot, H. Lewis, and B. N. Singh. Abolition of Holter monitor-detected silent myocardial ischemia after percutaneous transluminal coronary angioplasty. *J. Am. Coll. Cardiol., 10*:499 (1987).

30. B. R. Chaitman, U. Deligonul, M. J. Kern, and M. G. Vandormael. Prognostic importance of silent myocardial ischemia after coronary angioplasty (abstr). *Circulation, 76*(Suppl IV):78 (1987).

31. A. J. Raper, A. Hastillo, and W. J. Paulsen. The syndrome of sudden severe painless myocardial ischemia. *Am. Heart J., 107*:813 (1984).

32. D. Tzivoni, A. Gavish, J. Benhorin, S. Banai, A. Keren, and S. Stern. Day-to-day variability of myocardial ischemic episodes in coronary artery disease. *Am. J. Cardiol., 60*:1003 (1987).

33. E. G. Nabel, J. Barry, M. B. Rocco, S. Campbell, K. Mead, T. Fenton, E. J. Orav, and A. P. Selwyn. Variability of transient myocardial ischemia in ambulatory patients with coronary artery disease. *Circulation, 78*:60 (1988).

16
Surgical Treatment of Asymptomatic Coronary Artery Disease

Some investigators are adamantly against surgery in asymptomatic patients in general; others are in favor of it in very limited circumstances; yet others take a broader view. Unfortunately, many of the surgical series have no medical controls and, therefore, do not provide enough "light," merely "heat." Furthermore, in most instances, there is no documentation that these asymptomatic patients demonstrate myocardial ischemia preoperatively. Because surgical patients who are totally asymptomatic are small in number, they are usually combined in follow-up reports with patients who are asymptomatic following a myocardial infarction. In addition, at the present time, there is no specific surgical data on patients with

217

angina who have frequent asymptomatic episodes. For these reasons, I have not used the same subheadings as in other chapters but rather discuss the findings in terms of nonrandomized versus randomized studies. The latter are more numerous and will be discussed first.

I. NONRANDOMIZED STUDIES

Coronary bypass surgery in small numbers of asymptomatic patients has been performed at several hospitals (Table 1). Usually these patients are reported as part of a mixed series that includes asymptomatic and mildly symptomatic patients. The results involving the asymptomatic patients must then be dissected out from the main body of data. The study from the Seattle Heart Watch conducted by the University of Washington School of Medicine [1] is one such study. In this series, 114 patients were asymptomatic and 505 patients were mildly symptomatic. Prognosis was compared in medically and surgically treated patients. Even though the study was nonrandomized, it provides important data because the medically and surgically treated patients had similar baseline variables. The surgically treated patients had a lower mortality (via life-table analyses) then their medical counterparts, with the largest difference in survival seen in patients with triple-vessel disease and ejection fractions between 31 and 50% (Figure 1). This is the only nonrandomized study with control patients; it suggests a beneficial effect of surgery on mortality in asymptomatic

Table 1   Surgical Therapy in Asymptomatic Patients with Coronary Artery Disease[a] (Nonrandomized Studies)

Reporting institution	No. of patients	Perioperative mortality	Mean follow-up (mo)	Late mortality
Cleveland Clinic	17	0	75	0
University of Washington	392	15 (3.8%)	65	NA
Peter Bent Brigham	20	0	34	1 (5%)
Montreal Heart Institute	55	0	69	4 (7.3%)

NA = not available.
[a]All studies include patients with prior myocardial infarction. University of Washington, Peter Bent Brigham and Montreal Heart Institute studies also include patients with mild symptoms.

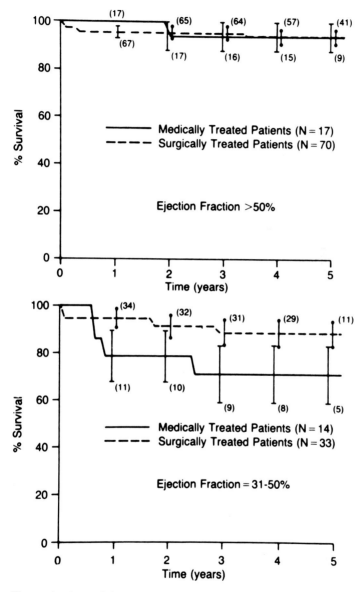

Figure 1 Actuarial survival curves comparing medically and surgically treated patients with three-vessel disease subgrouped according to ejection fraction. (From K. E. Hammermeister, T. A. DeRouen, and H. T. Dodge. *Circulation, 62*:98, 1980.)

patients. Because prognosis in patients with normal ejection fractions and mild or no symptoms appeared excellent, the authors did not feel anything but an enormous sample size would be sufficient to test the hypothesis that surgical therapy improves survival in that type of patients. Furthermore, there were too few asymptomatic patients with left main lesions for the authors to make any definite statements about treatment for that lesion, but they did feel that on the basis of their study, they would recommend surgery in patients with triple-vessel disease and moderate impairment of left ventricular function.

Table 2 Clinical Data on Patients with Minimal or no Angina Pectoris who Underwent CABG Surgery

Pt. no.	Age	MI	Angina pectoris	ETT Preop.	ETT Postop.	Diseased vessels (no.)	Grafts (no.)	Follow-up (mo)
1	49	+	−	0	0	2	2	80
2	54	−	−	+	−	LM	1	63
3	47	+	−	−	−	3	2	62 (1)
4	58	+	−	0	0	3	5	42
5	53	+	−	+	−	3	3	42
6	35	+	−	+	−	2	3	39
7	42	−	=	+	−	3	3	36
8	49	+	−	0	−	2	1	30
9	36	−	−	+	+	2	2	30
10	39	+	−	+	−	2	2	29
11	63	+	=	+	−	3	3	28
12	37	−	=	+	0	3	5	23
13	44	−	−	+	0	3	2	23
14	62	ı	ı	s	s	3	3	22
15	60	+	=	+	+	LM	3	22
16	43	+	=	−	0	2	3	21
17	55	−	=	+	−	LM	3	21
18	55	+	−	0	−	3	3	21
19	53	−	−	+	+	1	2	20
20	50	−	−	+	−	LM	2	19

CABG = coronary artery bypass surgery; ETT = exercise tolerance test; + = positive or present; − = negative or absent; = = mild; 0 = not done; D = late death; LM = left main coronary; MI = prior myocardial infarction.
Source: J. Wynne, L. H. Cohn, J. J. Collins, Jr., and P. F. Cohn. *Circulation, 58*(Suppl I):I-92, 1978.

In addition to this retrospective "matched" study from the University of Washington, there have also been several reports of surgical series without attempts to have control groups. Thus, Grondin et al. [2], at the Montreal Heart Institute, reported on 55 patients, 19 of whom were totally asymptomatic. Most patients had multivessel disease. There were four late deaths and seven late infarctions in the 69-month follow-up period, and despite the zero perioperative mortality, the authors questioned the

(a)

PREOPERATIVE

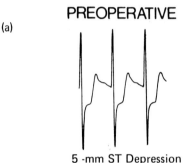

5 -mm ST Depression
Heart Rate: 145 beats/min
Duration of Exercise: 4.5 min

POSTOPERATIVE

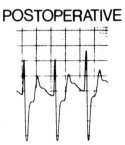

2-mm ST Depression
Heart Rate: 150 beats/min
Duration of Exercise: 10.5 min

(b)

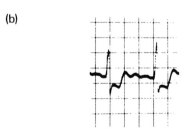

Positive 3-mm ST Depression
Heart Rate: 108 beats/min
Duration of Exercise: 7 min

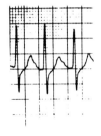

Negative
Heart Rate: 165 beats/min
Duration of Exercise: 10 min

Figure 2 Representative leads (V_4) from preoperative (left) and postoperative (right) exercise tolerance tests in two patients demonstrating improvement after surgery. (a) Improvement in degree of ST segment depression, and duration of exercise, and improvement in duration of exercise. (From J. Wynne, L. H. Cohn, J. J. Collins, Jr., and P. F. Cohn. *Circulation, 58*(Suppl 1):1-92, 1978.)

value of this type of prophylactic surgery. Thurer et al. [3] operated on 17 patients at the Cleveland Clinic who were asymptomatic after an infarction. Sixteen of the seventeen remained asymptomatic. The Peter Bent Brigham Hospital [4] experience was similar (Table 2). Twenty patients were studied, 14 of whom were totally asymptomatic. Six of these had sustained a prior myocardial infarction. This series was unique in that 16 patients had preoperative exercise tests, of which 14 demonstrated silent ischemia. The only death in this series occurred five years after surgery. There were 12 patients with both preoperative and postoperative exercise tests; in eight the test became completely normal, while in the other four, less of an ischemic response was observed compared to the preoperative test. Examples of these exercise tests are depicted in Figure 2. Schnellbacher et al. [5] recently reported that in a series of 22 surgically treated totally asymptomatic patients, all of them did well clinically and showed reduction or absence of ST depression on exercise tests. Fitzgibbon et al. [6] reported on a series of 723 consecutive patients operated on between 1971 and 1979. The authors separated the 118 patients who had no angina three years prior to the study from the 605 who had angina. No important differences in survival between the patients was noted.

II. RANDOMIZED STUDIES

The multicenter Coronary Artery Surgery Study (CASS) [7-9] has provided additional data both for and against surgical intervention. Unlike the Seattle report, this was a randomized study, but one with certain qualifying features. First, many patients had sustained myocardial infarctions. Second, they all had undergone coronary arteriography prior to randomization. Third, patients with left main lesions or ejection fractions less than 0.35 were excluded. Fourth, although only patients with no angina or mild angina (Class I and II NYHA) were included, many patients required medication to attain this pain-free or mild-pain classification. From the original 16,626 patients who underwent coronary arteriography at 15 sites from 1974 to 1979, 780 patients with stable ischemic heart disease were randomized to medical or surgical therapy; 390 patients were in each group. With only one exception, there were no statistically significant differences in survival in patients receiving medical versus surgical therapy. The exception was the triple-vessel disease subgroup with >0.50 ejection fraction [8,9]. As discussed earlier in Chapter 12, the existence of high-risk patients within the three-vessel disease subgroup with normal left ventricular function can be verified only when additional tests beside

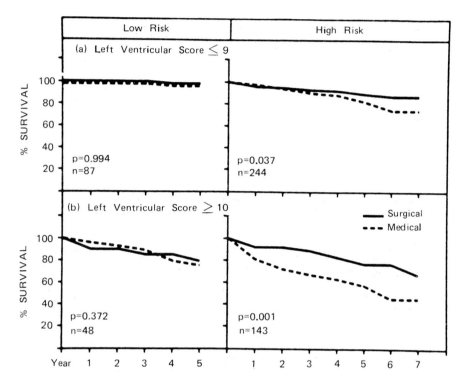

Figure 3 Cumulative survival rates in the surgical (solid line) and medical (dotted line) groups among patients with three-vessel coronary disease stratified by the left ventricular score according to the exercise risk classification. A lower risk subgroup comprised patients with less than 1mm of ST-segment depression and a final exercise stage of 3 or higher, whereas a higher risk subset consisted of patients with 1mm or greater of ST-segment depression and a final exercise stage of 1 or less. (From D. A. Weiner, T. J. Ryan, C. H. McCabe, B. R. Chaitman, L. T. Sheffield, L. D. Fisher, and F. Tristani. *Am. J. Cardiol., 60*:262, 1987.)

the coronary angiogram and left ventriculogram are performed. For example, risk clarification is enhanced when the exercise test is employed. The best surgical candidates amongst patients with *normal* left ventricular function can now be identified (Figure 3) [10].

A smaller randomized trial of medical versus surgical management was carried out at Green Lane Hospital in New Zealand [11]. One hundred patients who were asymptomatic after a myocardial infarction were followed for a mean period of four and a half years. Annual mortality was 2% in both groups. These patients had at least two infarcts and had to survive at least two months postinfarction to be included in the randomization process. The patients—most with extensive coronary artery disease—again had a surprisingly low annual mortality and most were not on beta-blocking agents. This makes it difficult for surgical survival to be "better." Furthermore, of the four surgical deaths, one was from noncardiac causes and one died while awaiting surgery. This study has been criticized because of the 2-month lag before randomization began; it is in this period that most of the medical deaths occur.

III. CONCLUSIONS

After reviewing this data, what is one to conclude? Should surgery be withheld from asymptomatic patients, as some argue [12]? Or is it indicated in selected instances such as patients with left main or triple-vessel disease, and left ventricular dysfunction, as others maintain [13,14]? In my view, it is the latter opinion that provides the best guidelines at present. Patients with less extensive disease can be managed with medical therapy and, at times, with angioplasty.

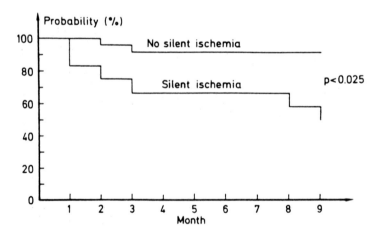

Figure 4 Kaplan-Meier curves of cumulative probabilities for cardiac events during a 9-month postoperative follow-up in 12 patients (group 1) with silent ischemia and 24 patients (group 2) without silent ischemia during ambulatory monitoring. (From K. Egstrup. *Am. J. Cardiol.,* *61*:248, 1988).

Although survival figures are obviously a "hard" end-point, evaluation of patients after surgery must also consider whether ischemia has been relieved. This is difficult to evaluate subjectively but it can be done with objective tests of myocardial function such as exercise tests and ambulatory ECG monitoring. The latter represents a new approach that may be especially useful in evaluating patients with both symptomatic and asymptomatic episodes [15]. As with exercise testing, residual ischemic episodes without pain may be demonstrated. They are an adverse marker for future cardiac events (Figure 4) [16].

REFERENCES

1. K. E. Hammermeister, T. A. DeRouen, and H. T. Dodge. Effect of coronary surgery on survival in asymptomatic and minimally symptomatic patients. *Circulation, 62*:98 (1980).

2. C. M. Grondin, J. G. Kretz, P. Vouhe, J. F. Tubau, L. Compeau, and M. G. Bourassa. Prophylactic coronary artery grafting in patients with few or no symptoms. *Ann. Thorac. Surg., 28*:113 (1978).

3. R. L. Thurer, B. W. Lytle, D. M. Cosgrove, and F. D. Loop. Asymptomatic coronary artery disease managed by myocardial revascularization: Results at 5 years. *Circulation, 61*(Suppl 1):I-92 (1978).

4. J. Wynne, L. H. Cohn, J. J. Collins, Jr., and P. F. Cohn. Myocardial revascularization in patients with multivessel coronary artery disease and minimal angina pectoris. *Circulation, 58*(Suppl I):I-92 (1978).

5. K. Schnellbacher, K. C. Droste, and H. Roskamm. Medical and surgical therapy of patients with asymptomatic ischemia. In *Silent Ischemia: Current Concepts in Detection and Management.* (T. von Arnim and A. Maseri, eds.), Steinkopff, Darmstadt, 1987, p. 133.

6. G. M. Fitzgibbon, J. R. Buron, and W. J. Keon. Aortocoronary bypass surgery in "asymptomatic" patients with coronary artery disease. In *Silent Myocardial Ischemia* (W. Rutishauser and H. Roskamm, eds.), Springer-Verlag, Berlin, 1984, pp. 180-193.

7. CASS Principal Investigators and their Associates. Coronary Artery Surgery Study (CASS): A randomized trial of coronary artery bypass surgery: Survival data. *Circulation, 68*:939 (1983).

8. E. Passamani, K. B. Davis, M. J. Gillespie, T. Killip, and the CASS Principal Investigators and their associates. A randomized trial of coronary bypass surgery. Survival of patients with a low ejection fraction. *N. Engl. J. Med., 312*: 1665 (1985).

9. D. A. Weiner, T. J. Ryan, C. H. McCabe, S. Luk, B. R. Chaitman, L. T. Sheffield, L. D. Fisher, and F. E. Tristani. Comparison of coronary artery

bypass surgery and medical therapy in patient with exercise-induced silent myocardial ischemia. *J. Am. Coll. Cardiol. 12*:595 (1988).

10. D. A. Weiner, T. J. Ryan, C. H. McCabe, B. R. Chaitman, L. T. Sheffield, L. D. Fisher, and F. Tristani. Value of exercise testing in determining the risk classification and the response to coronary artery bypass grafting in three-vessel coronary artery disease: A report from the Coronary Artery Surgery Study (CASS) Registry. *Am. J. Cardiol., 60*:262 (1987).

11. R. M. Norris, T. M. Agnes, P. W. T. Brandt, K. J. Graham, D. G. Jill, A. R. Kerr, J. B. Lowe, A. H. G. Roche, R. M. L. Whitlock, and B. G. Barrett-Boyes. Coronary surgery after a recurrent myocardial infarction: Progress of a trial comparing surgical with nonsurgical management for asymptomatic patients with advanced coronary disease. *Circulation, 63*:785 (1981).

12. A. Selzer and K. Cohn. Asymptomatic coronary artery disease and coronary bypass surgery. *Am. J. Cardiol., 39*:614 (1977).

13. K. M. Kent, D. R. Rosing, C. J. Ewels, L. Kipson, R. Bonow, and S. E. Epstein. Prognosis of asymptomatic or mildly symptomatic patients with coronary artery disease. *Am. J. Cardiol., 49*:1823 (1982).

14. S. E. Epstein, A. A. Quyyumi, and R. O. Bonow. Myocardial ischemia—Silent or symptomatic. *N. Engl. J. Med., 318*:1039 (1988).

15. P. Ribeiro, M. Shea, J. E. Deanfield, C. M. Oakley, R. Sapsford, T. Jones, R. Walesby, and A. P. Selwyn. Different mechanisms for the relief of angina after coronary bypass surgery: Physiological versus anatomical assessment. *Br. Heart J., 52*:502 (1984).

16. K. Egstrup. Asymptomatic myocardial ischemia as a predictor of cardiac events after coronary artery bypass grafting for stable angina pectoris. *Am. J. Cardiol., 61*:248 (1988).

VI
FUTURE DIRECTIONS

17

Silent Myocardial Ischemia and Silent Myocardial Infarction

What Issues Remain to Be Resolved?

In the past 3 years there has been a considerable increase in the amount of information available to physicians concerning silent coronary artery disease. Some of the issues raised in the 1986 (first) edition of this book have been clarified, others have not and new issues have emerged. The 1986 workshop sponsored by the National Institutes of Health (NIH) helped to focus attention on many of these problems.

I. SILENT MYOCARDIAL ISCHEMIA

Present lines of investigation have included emphasis on the pathophysiologic mechanisms of silent myocardial ischemia. In particular, the work

229

of Droste and Roskamm [1] on pain thresholds seems confirmed by the work of Glazier et al. [2]. Thus, there appears to be an alteration in the somatic pain mechanisms in some individuals. The basis of this neurologic or humoral abnormality remains unclear. Future lines of investigation should explore this. If there is an alteration in somatic or cardiac pain perception, is this alteration found only in individuals with Type 1 or Type 2 silent ischemia? Do anginal patients with episodes of silent ischemia (Type 3 patients) have a different pathophysiologic mechanism, i.e., less myocardium at jeopardy? The coronary balloon angioplasty data seems to suggest this is *not* the case in the Type 3 patient, but better techniques to quantitate the amount of ischemic myocardium—during both symptomatic and asymptomatic episodes—will be necessary for this hypothesis to be confirmed. The widespread use of angioplasty now offers a safe way of producing transient transmural ischemia in an "approved" manner and should lead to even more data for comparisons of symptomatic versus asymptomatic episodes. As far as the triggering mechanism that actually precipitates the ischemic event, exciting new research into endothelial factors and platelet aggregation may be able to resolve this issue—for both painful and painless episodes.

Estimates of the prevalence of the various types of silent myocardial ischemia are more reliable now that more centers report data in Type 2 and Type 3 patients. While it will be difficult logistically and financially for one center in the United States to duplicate Erikssen's Norwegian study [3], it would certainly be interesting to see the results of this kind of diagnostic approach in Type 1 persons in a multicentered study in the United States. But the cost of this kind of study still argues against its feasibility, as do the financial and ethical questions of confirmatory coronary angiography. It is much simpler to obtain hard data on the prevalence of silent ischemia in asymptomatic *postinfarction* patients. The frequency of exercise testing (and Holter monitor studies) in this subgroup make it a fertile source of information and several groups have begun multicenter collaborations. Similarly, Holter monitoring in angina patients should provide reliable figures on the prevalence of Type 3 silent ischemia. The nationwide Nifedipine-Total Ischemia Awareness Program (TIAP) is an example of what can be done [4]. We can expect other similar studies to soon present their own data.

Studies that establish the prevalence of the three types of silent myocardial ischemia can also be used to obtain more natural history data, as Erikssen has done in his investigations. Similar *prospective* studies in Types 2 and 3 patients are underway. Holter monitors appear reliable enough to provide such data. The next generation (the real-time devices) are constantly being improved to yield reliable ST segment recording. Such prospective studies are essential for making intelligent management decisions. But management decisions will require more than natural history data. They will require interventional arms. Here is where the circulatory dynamics of the ischemic episodes come into play. Is there truly a vasospastic component and, therefore, are nitrates and calcium antagonists better suited for this syndrome than beta-adrenergic blocking agents? Should the latter be used only in exertion-induced episodes? Early results suggest a wider role for the beta-blockers. Finally, what happens to the subgroup of asymptomatic patients with left main and/or three-vessel disease? Are they truly as susceptible to sudden death and massive infarcts as suggested by the Norwegian data, or are they always warned by symptoms and their course more benign [5]? How should they be treated? Medically? Surgically? [5]

II. SILENT MYOCARDIAL INFARCTION AND SUDDEN CARDIAC DEATH

We have made important strides in documenting the prevalence of silent myocardial infarction; the Framingham Study [6] is a good example of this kind of prospective investigation. Again, as in silent myocardial ischemia, we are not sure why nondiabetic individuals do not experience pain with their infarcts. Even though this is "softer" data (because physicians in general do not observe the infarct as we do the transient episodes of silent ischemia), there is still much that can be learned about these patients. Are they also experiencing episodes of silent ischemia? What is the incidence of recurrent silent infarctions? These questions remain as unclear now as in 1986. With widespread Holter monitoring, we should be documenting many more of these infarctions and their arrhythmic complications as they occur, which leads us to the last and perhaps most important issue.

What is the relationship of silent ischemia and infarctions to sudden cardiac death? Some evidence from Erikssen's study [4] supports this link, but more data are necessary. There are many aspects of sudden cardiac death that remain to be unraveled, but one aspect of this syndrome is particularly fascinating. Are these individuals experiencing silent ischemia prior to their demise? The study by Sharma et al. [7] suggest that this is so. To take survivors of cardiac death and systematically test them for silent ischemia requires a concerted effort from several centers and by definition, we can only investigate survivors. Is this somehow a skewered population? This is one question we may never be able to answer, but the public health consequences are enormous.

REFERENCES

1. C. Droste and H. Roskamm. Experimental pain measurements in patients with asymptomatic myocardial ischemia. *J. Am. Coll. Cardiol., 1*:940 (1983).

2. J. J. Glazier, S. Chierchia, M. J. Brown, and A. Maseri. Importance of generalized defective perception of painful stimuli as a cause of silent myocardial ischemia in chronic stable angina pectoris. *Am. J. Cardiol., 58*:667 (1986).

3. J. Erikssen and E. Thaulow. Follow-up of patients with asymptomatic myocardial ischemia. In *Silent Myocardial Ischemia* (W. Rutishauser and H. Roskamm, eds.), Springer-Verlag, Berlin, 1984, pp. 156-164.

4. P. F. Cohn, G. W. Vetrovec, R. Nesto, and the Total Ischemia Awareness Program Investigators. A national survey of painful and painless myocardial ischemia: The Total Ischemia Awareness Program (preliminary report) (abstr). *J. Am. Coll. Cardiol., 11*:203A (1988).

5. S. E. Epstein, A. A. Quyyumi, and R. A. Bonow. Myocardial ischemia—Silent or symptomatic. *N. Engl. J. Med., 318*:1039 (1988).

6. W. B. Kannel and R. D. Abbott. Incidence and prognosis of unrecognized myocardial infarction: An update on the Framingham Study. *N. Engl. J. Med., 311*:1144 (1984).

7. B. Sharma, R. Asinger, G. S. Francis, M. Hodges, and R. P. Wyeth. Demonstration of exercise-induced ischemia without angina in survivors of out-of-hospital ventricular fibrillation. *Am. J. Cardiol., 59*:740 (1981).

Index

A

Ambulatory electrocardiographic
(Holter) monitoring, 103-120,
177, 178, 180, 205, 207, 210

Angina pectoris
circulatory dynamics of, 42-45
pathophysiology of, compared
to silent myocardial ischemia,
42-53
prognosis of, compared to silent
myocardial ischemia, 177-180
treatment of, compared to silent
myocardial ischemia, 206-211,
217-225
unstable, prognostic significance
of painless episodes, 180

Apoprotein B, as marker for asymptomatic coronary artery disease,
97

Arrhythmias
exericse-induced, 130
ventricular, as indicators
of asymptomatic coronary
artery disease, 100, 186-
191

Arteriography, coronary
cardiac catheterization and, *see*
Cardiac catheterization
findings of, in coronary artery
patients with and without
angina, 155-158, 171-180,
187, 188
indications for, 152-155